T0384366

Management of Snoring
and Obstructive Sleep Apnea

D.S. Deenadayal
Vyshanavi Bommakanti

Management of Snoring and Obstructive Sleep Apnea

A Practical Guide

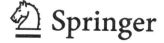 Springer

D.S. Deenadayal
DR.Deenadayals ENT Care Centre
Secunderabad, Telangana, India

Vyshanavi Bommakanti
Shenoy Hospitals
Secunderabad, Telangana, India

ISBN 978-981-16-6619-3   ISBN 978-981-16-6620-9   (eBook)
https://doi.org/10.1007/978-981-16-6620-9

This Springer imprint is published by the registered company Springer Nature Singapore Pte Ltd. The registered company address is: 152 Beach Road, #21-01/04 Gateway East, Singapore 189721, Singapore

Contents

List of Figures

List of Tables

Introduction

The term "sleep disordered breathing" refers to a range of conditions that result in abnormal breathing during sleep.

Sleep-disordered breathing (SDB) is a continuum of disorders, which ranges as shown below, depending on the level of obstruction (Fig. 1.1).

The event of snoring indicates some degrees of airway obstruction. While snoring indicates a partial airway obstruction, apnea indicates a complete airway obstruction.

Many OSA patients remain undiagnosed or remain reluctant to seek treatment for their condition as they are unaware of the newer treatment options available.

Obstructive sleep apnea (OSA) is characterized by episodes of partial or complete obstruction of the upper airway during sleep, thus interrupting (apnea) or reducing (hypopnea) the flow of air.

These cycles of apnea/hypopnea which repeat several times an hour, result in fragmented and disturbed sleep.

The upper airway, particularly the oropharynx and hypopharynx, is the region where most obstructive processes leading to OSA occur.

In the age group of 30–35 years, around 20% of men and 5% of women snore. By the age of 60, this percentage increases to 60% in men and 40% in women [1].

Snoring is three times more common in obese individuals [2] and is a terrible marital and social problem.

OSAS has a negative impact on the health and behavior of millions of people throughout the world.

It is also an independent risk factor for many diseases, such as hypertension, heart failure, heart attack, cardiovascular events, and arrhythmias.

Today, sleep-disordered breathing is recognized as a distinct clinical entity that requires to be evaluated and treated.

In order to ensure the holistic treatment of a patient suffering from sleep-related disorders, different specialists, namely a pulmonologist, a neurologist, an orthodontist, and an otolaryngologist, are required to collaborate and work as a team.

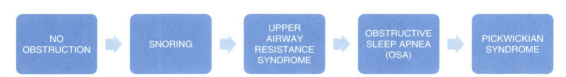

Fig. 1.1 Continuum of sleep-disordered breathing

References

1. Bonsignore MR, Saaresranta T, Riha RL, Riha R, Bonsignore M. Sex differences in obstructive sleep apnoea. Eur Respir Rev [Internet]. 2019 Dec 31;28(154):190030. [cited 2021 Feb 19]. Available from: https://err.ersjournals.com/content/28/154/190030.

2. Krupp K, Wilcox M, Srinivas A, Srinivas V, Madhivanan P, Bastida E. Snoring is associated with obesity among middle aged slum-dwelling women in Mysore, India. Lung India [Internet]. 2020;37(3):210. [cited 2021 Feb 19]. Available from: https://www.ncbi.nlm.nih.gov/pmc/articles/PMC7353948/.

2.1 Evolution of SDB

Snoring and the subsequent diagnosis of obstructive sleep apnea (OSA) was a life-threatening medical condition with no available treatment until the late twentieth century.

In the early reports of the 50s, obstructive sleep apnea was termed as an uncommon disease. However, a few years later, in the 70s, hundreds of cases were reported. It was in 1975 that Carroll et al. described the differences between the Pickwickian syndrome and OSA [1].

Thereafter, since the last two decades, there has been a paradigm shift in the diagnosis and management of OSA.

2.2 Evolution of an Otolaryngologist in the Treatment of OSA

Until the early 2000s, the most common specialists who were involved in the treatment of SDB were a neurologist or a pulmonologist. Otolaryngologists played a small role in definitive treatment in sleep medicine. Since neurologists are trained to read an EEG, they could interpret the polysomnography data with ease and the pulmonologist displayed an expertise in the use of positive airway pressure therapy, thus making them the primary physicians in the area of sleep medicine until recent times.

Over the years, otolaryngologists have been trained for upper airway surgeries. However, they were still not considered primary physicians in sleep medicine and their opinion was sought only if surgical intervention was deemed necessary by the primary care physician.

However, today, otolaryngology is a specialty that deals with both surgical and non-surgical treatments of the upper airway. Otolaryngologists, unlike many other specialists, hold the expertise to obtain a thorough history, to do a proper clinical examination, and to assess dysfunction and disorders of the upper airway. They do not wait for patients with sleep disorders to be referred to them by other treatment providers of sleep medicine.

2.3 Evolution of Diagnosis

There has been a remarkable evolution in the diagnostic tools available for screening and diagnosing patients with SDB. Before the advent of sleep laboratories, most research focused on the treatment of snoring. It was speculated that the sounds produced while snoring were due to the vibrations from the epiglottis, velum, cheeks, or nostrils and this was later on confirmed with a nasopharyngoscope. A few decades ago, OSA was considered a rare entity, solely because there were no diagnostic tools available. But today, there are numerous diagnostic tools ranging from

D. S. Deenadayal, V. Bommakanti, *Management of Snoring and Obstructive Sleep Apnea*, https://doi.org/10.1007/978-981-16-6620-9_2

polysomnography, drug induced sleep endoscopy, fiberoptic laryngopharyngoscopy, dynamic MRI, and so on.

This availability of various investigative methods with better sensitivity and specificity has increased the diagnosis of patients with sleep-disordered breathing.

2.4 Evolution of Treatment

Until two decades, PAP therapy was considered to be the only treatment option for patients with OSA. Sullivan et al. in 1981, first introduced the use of CPAP in the treatment of snoring and OSA in adults and their results showed a complete cessation of upper airway obstruction resulting in a comfortable night's sleep [2]. Although effective, it was found to be cumbersome and not many could even access a CPAP machine when required. This led to a quest for finding other alternative options, like surgery, for the treatment of obstructive sleep apnea.

In the 1970s, a tracheostomy became the standard approach in the treatment of Pickwickian syndrome, OSA, and severe daytime somnolence with associated hypertension and cardiac electrophysiological changes [1].

It was not until 1976, that Ikematsu first described an uvulopalatopharyngoplasty (UPPP) as an alternative surgical treatment of "snoring," with a reported cure rate of 81% [1]. The only other surgical procedure for OSA treatment was a permanent tracheostomy.

UPPP was introduced in the USA as an alternative to a permanent tracheostomy by Fujita in 1981 [1]. This appeared to be the first of multiple procedures that used the same concept for the reconstruction of the soft palate.

Since then, multiple surgical approaches and combinations of approaches have surfaced, with variable success rates.

There has also been a vast change in the surgical techniques used. Initially more radical procedures like a tracheostomy and radical resection of tissues for uvulopalatopharyngoplasty were performed. In the more recent times, however, more conservative surgeries are preferred with minimal tissue resection being the aim of OSA surgeries.

The surgical techniques have changed from radical surgery to conservative surgery, from excision of tissue to reshaping and remodeling the tissue of the airway. Currently, surgeries for patients with OSA are now tailor made and modified based on the level of obstruction that has been found. Single surgeries or multistep surgeries may be performed based on the level of obstruction.

Recent advances include palatal implants and hypoglossal nerve stimulation that reduce the occurrence of obstructive sleep apnea by electrically stimulating the hypoglossal nerve of the tongue.

2.5 Evolution in Technology

PAP Devices: The only device available for treatment of OSA until recently was a CPAP. At present there are also other devices like a Bilevel Positive airway pressure and servo ventilation depending on the necessity.

Surgical tools: With various technological advances in the field of medicine, LASER which was being used in the past for the vaporization of the soft palate is not being used anymore.

Recent introduction of devices like radiofrequency, coblation, and robotics in the treatment of OSA have increased precision in surgeries and reduced complications, thus making OSA surgeries safe and effective.

Despite all the advances in OSA surgery in the last few decades, there is no single treatment option that will be successful for all patients. A treatment plan that best caters to the needs of the patient must be devised and followed.

References

1. Yaremchuk K, Garcia-Rodriguez L. The history of sleep surgery [Internet]. Adv Oto-Rhino-Laryngol. 2017;80:17–21. Available from: https://www.karger.com/Article/Pdf/470683.

2. Sullivan CE, Berthon-Jones M, Issa FG, Eves L. Reversal of obstructive sleep Apnoea by continuous positive airway pressure applied through the nares. Lancet. 1981 Apr 18;317(8225):862–5.

Co-morbidities are the presence of one or more additional conditions co-occurring with a primary condition. Several studies have reported a high prevalence of co-morbidities in OSA patients and the number of co-morbidities seen is found to be directly proportional to the severity of the OSA.

3.1 Effects of Obstructive Sleep Apnea (Fig. 3.1)

3.2 Obstructive Sleep Apnea and Systemic Hypertension

OSA is highly prevalent in patients with hypertension. About 50% of patients with HTN have concomitant OSA [1] (Fig. 3.2).

Blood pressure normally follows a diurnal pattern such that the average nocturnal systolic blood pressure is >10% lower than during the daytime. This physiological nocturnal BP decrease (dipping pattern) is altered in patients with OSA. The loss of this nocturnal dipping blood pressure pattern, in both normotensive and hypertensive subjects, is associated with a worse cardiovascular prognosis [1].

Raised blood pressure in OSA patients results in hypertensive target organ damage which further leads to conditions such as hypertensive heart disease (left ventricular hypertrophy, diastolic dysfunction, left atrial enlargement), silent cerebral disease (silent cerebral infarcts, white matter disease), and microalbuminuria.

3.3 Obstructive Sleep Apnea and Cardiovascular Diseases

- With the recognition of hypoxemia that could occur with OSA, there is now a growing interest in the cardiovascular consequences of sleep disorders.
- There is a 2.4-times increased likelihood of having OSA with underlying heart failure [2] (Fig. 3.3).

3.3.1 OSA and Sudden Cardiac Death

The prevalence of sleep-disordered breathing in patients with coronary artery disease is about two times greater than in patients without.

Severe OSA was associated with an increased risk of fatal and non-fatal cardiac events [3] (Fig. 3.4).

© The Author(s), under exclusive license to Springer Nature Singapore Pte Ltd. 2022
D. S. Deenadayal, V. Bommakanti, *Management of Snoring and Obstructive Sleep Apnea*,
https://doi.org/10.1007/978-981-16-6620-9_3

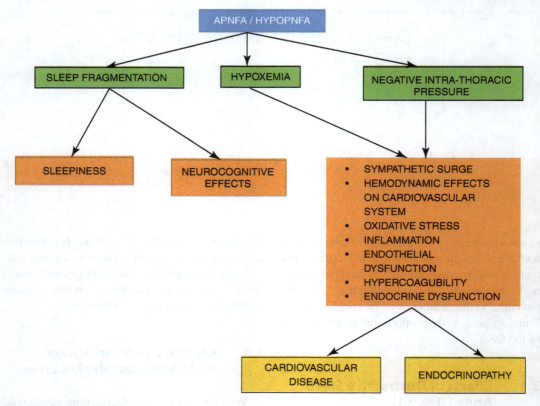

Fig. 3.1 Effects of OSA

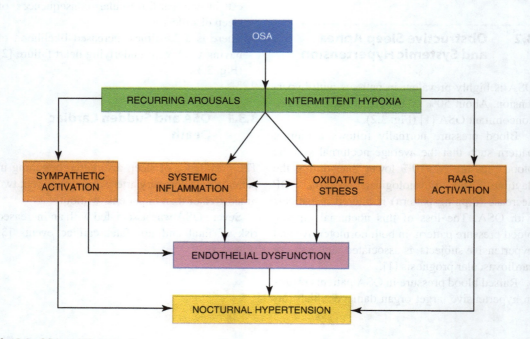

Fig. 3.2 OSA and Hypertension

Fig. 3.3 OSA and cardiovascular diseases

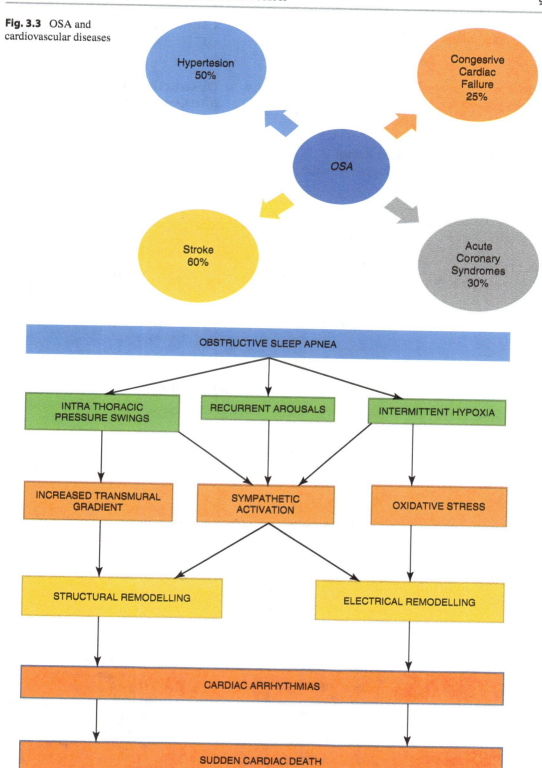

Fig. 3.4 OSA and Sudden Cardiac Death

3.3.2 Obstructive Sleep Apnea and Arrhythmias

Over 50% of patients with OSA have nocturnal arrhythmias that increase in frequency in relation to increases in AHI and severity of hypoxemia [4].

3.3.3 Obstructive Sleep Apnea and Pulmonary Hypertension (PHT)

Acute pulmonary hemodynamic changes during obstructive apnea have been well defined.

Nocturnal desaturation, however, was linked with daytime PHT [5] (Fig. 3.5).

3.4 Obstructive Sleep Apnea and Central Nervous System

3.4.1 Obstructive Sleep Apnea and Cerebrovascular Stroke

Patients with severe sleep apnea are at a 3 to four-fold increased risk of stroke but there is no definitive evidence that OSA is an independent risk factor for stroke [6, 7] (Fig. 3.6).

Fig. 3.5 OSA and Pulmonary Hypertension

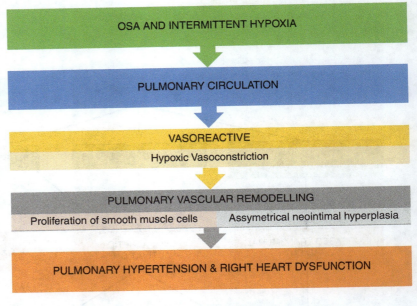

Fig. 3.6 OSA and Stroke

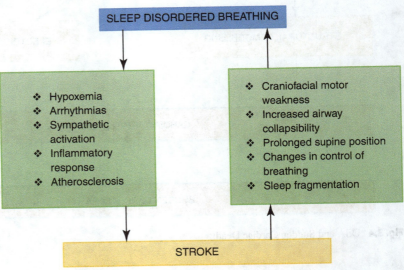

Patients with OSA demonstrate variable degrees of cognitive, emotional, and performance deficits. OSA is increasingly being recognized as one of the potentially modifiable risk factors for dementia [8].

REM sleep is suggested to play a role in recalibrating the sensitivity and specificity of the brain's response to positive and negative emotional events [9].

Various mental health issues, such as affective disorders, emotional instability, depression, and aggravation of post-traumatic stress disorder are some co-morbidities commonly associated with OSA [10].

3.4.2 Obstructive Sleep Apnea and Metabolic Diseases

Sleep apnea results in intermittent hypoxia and sleep fragmentation, which in turn leads to and exacerbates obesity and type 2 diabetes by increasing sympathetic activity, oxidative stress, inflammation, and lipolysis [11]. Metabolic disease can lead to, or exacerbate sleep apnea through weight-dependent and physiology-dependent mechanisms. Thus, the relationship between obstructive sleep apnea and metabolic disease is bidirectional [11] (Fig. 3.7).

3.4.3 Metabolic Pathways Linking OSA to Type 2 Diabetes

Untreated OSA in diabetic patients is associated with increased prevalence of neuropathy, peripheral arterial disease, diabetic retinopathy, and diabetic nephropathy [12].

It must be understood that, treatment of OSA may or may not improve glycemic control in diabetic patients but it will help to prevent severe consequences of diabetes [12].

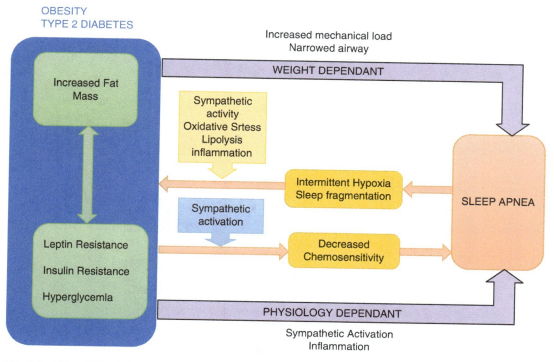

Fig. 3.7 OSA and Metabolic Disorders

3.5   Obstructive Sleep Apnea and Respiratory Diseases

Both OSA and chronic obstructive pulmonary disease (COPD) overlap and may occur in the same patient [12] (Fig. 3.8).

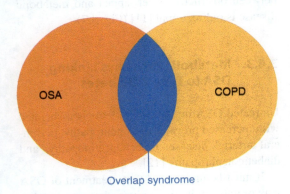

Fig. 3.8 OSA and COPD

Studies have also shown that OSA is more common in asthmatics. There are studies confirming the association of OSA with asthma and obesity, especially in women [12].

3.6   Obstructive Sleep Apnea and Reproductive System

Reproductive hormones may modify sleep patterns and this relationship is bidirectional, i.e. the disruption of sleep patterns may also alter the profile of reproductive hormone secretion [13].

Thus, OSA may result in infertility, low libido, erectile dysfunction, impotence, and azoospermia [14, 15] (Figs. 3.9 and 3.10).

The co-morbidities associated with OSA are [16] (Table 3.1):

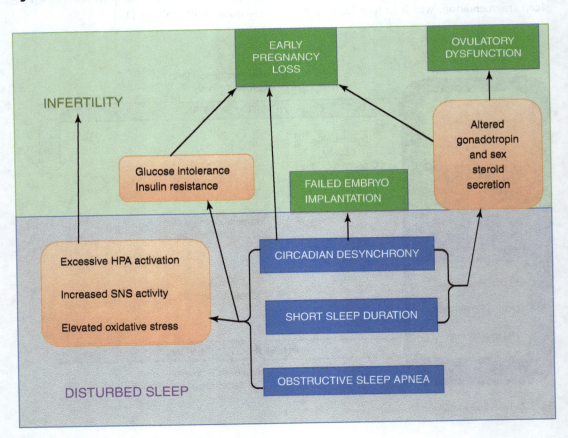

Fig. 3.9 OSA and Female reproductive system

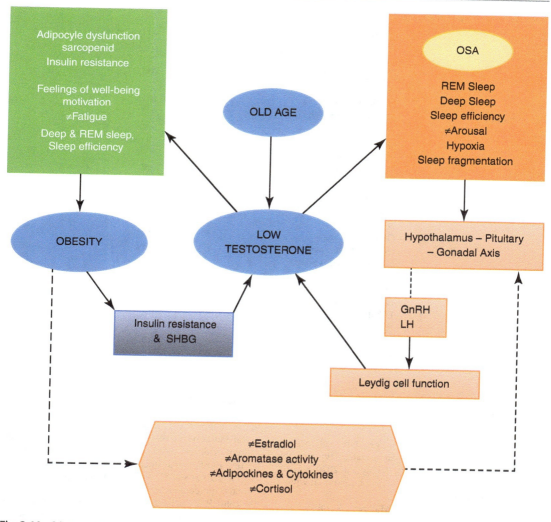

Fig. 3.10 OSA and Male reproductive System

3.6.1   Co-Morbidities and Consequences of Pediatric OSA

The co-morbidities associated with pediatric OSA are described in chap. 13. Here we describe, in brief, the consequences of OSA in the pediatric population.

Neuropsychological sequelae: They include cognitive deficits, behavioral abnormalities, increased daytime sleepiness, hyperactivity and/or attention deficit hyperactivity disorder (ADHD), depression, and poor quality of life.

Cardiovascular sequelae: They include ventricular hypertrophy (right, left, biventricular), pulmonary hypertension, Cor-pulmonale, elevated blood pressure, and autonomic instability.

Metabolic sequelae: OSA in pediatric population has been known to affect growth caused by a decrease in the serum insulin-like growth factor (IGF) and it has also been known to be associated with metabolic syndromes.

Craniofacial changes: These children have high arched palates, due to chronic mouth breathing, crowding of teeth, and other craniofacial changes, putting them at risk for adult OSA.

Table 3.1 Co-morbidities associated with OSA

Category	Condition	Prevalence [%]
Cardiac	– Hypertension/resistant hypertension – Congestive heart failure – Ischemic heart disease – Atrial fibrillation – Dysrhythmias	63-83% 76% 38% 49% 58%
Respiratory	– Pulmonary hypertension – Asthma	77% 18%
Neurologic	– Stroke – Worsening of epilepsy	71-90%
Metabolic	– Type 2 diabetes mellitus – Metabolic syndrome – Morbid obesity	36% 50% 50-90%
Others	– Gastroesophageal reflux – Nocturia – Glaucoma – Head and neck cancer – Traffic accidents – Glaucoma – Snoring spouse syndrome – Diminished libido – PCOD – Renal failure – Hypothyroidism – GERD	60% 48% 20% 76%

References

1. Konecny T, Kara T, Somers VK. Obstructive sleep apnea and hypertension: an update. Hypertension [Internet]. 2014 Feb;63(2):203. [cited 2020 Sep 6]. Available from: https://www.ncbi.nlm.nih.gov/pmc/articles/PMC4249687/.

2. Kohli P, Balachandran JS, Malhotra A. Obstructive sleep apnea and the risk for cardiovascular disease [Internet]. Curr Atheroscler Rep. 2011;13:138–46. NIH Public Access. [cited 2020 Sep 6]. Available from: https://www.ncbi.nlm.nih.gov/pmc/articles/PMC4332589/?report=abstract.

3. Jean-Louis G, Brown CD, Zizi F, Ogedegbe G, Boutin-Foster C, Gorga J, et al. Cardiovascular disease risk reduction with sleep apnea treatment [Internet]. Expert Rev Cardiovasc Ther. 2010;8:995–1005. Expert Reviews Ltd. [cited 2021 Feb 19]. Available from: https://www.ncbi.nlm.nih.gov/pmc/articles/PMC4234108/.

4. Gonzaga C, Bertolami A, Bertolami M, Amodeo C, Calhoun D. Obstructive sleep apnea, hypertension and cardiovascular diseases. J Hum Hypertens [Internet]. 2015;29(12):705–12. Available from: http://www.ncbi.nlm.nih.gov/pubmed/25761667

5. Lattimore JDL, Celermajer DS, Wilcox I. Obstructive sleep apnea and cardiovascular disease. J Am Coll Cardiol [Internet]. 2003 May 7;41(9):1429–37. [cited 2020 Sep 8]. Available from: https://www.onlinejacc.org/content/41/9/1429.

6. McNicholas WT, Bonsignore MR. Sleep apnoea as an independent risk for cardiovascular disease: current evidence, basic mechanisms and research priorities. Eur Respir J [Internet]. 2007 Jan 1;29(1):156–78. [cited 2020 Sep 8]. Available from: https://erj.ersjournals.com/content/29/1/156.

7. Kohli P, Balachandran JS, Malhotra A. Obstructive sleep apnea and the risk for cardiovascular disease. Curr Atheroscler Rep. 2011;13:138–46.

8. Cross NE, Memarian N, Duffy SL, Paquola C, LaMonica H, D'Rozario A, et al. Structural brain correlates of obstructive sleep apnoea in older adults at risk for dementia. Eur Respir J [Internet]. 2018 Jul 1;52(1):1800740. [cited 2020 Sep 8]. Available from: https://doi.org/10.1183/13993003.00740-2018.

9. Goldstein AN, Walker MP. The role of sleep in emotional brain function [Internet]. Annu Rev Clin Psychol. 2014;10:679–708. Annual Reviews Inc. [cited 2020 Sep 8]. Available from: https://www.ncbi.nlm.nih.gov/pmc/articles/PMC4286245/?report=abstract.

10. Gupta MA, Simpson FC. Obstructive sleep apnea and psychiatric disorders: a systematic review. J Clin Sleep Med. 2015;11:165–75. American Academy of Sleep Medicine

11. Framnes SN, Arble DM. The bidirectional relationship between obstructive sleep apnea and metabolic

disease [Internet]. Front Endocrinol. 2018;9:440. Frontiers Media S.A. [cited 2020 Sep 8]. Available from: https://www.ncbi.nlm.nih.gov/pmc/articles/PMC6087747/?report=abstract.

12. Bonsignore MR, Baiamonte P, Mazzuca E, Castrogiovanni A, Marrone O. Obstructive sleep apnea and comorbidities: a dangerous liaison [internet]. Multidiscip Respir Med. 2019;14:1–12. [cited 2020 Sep 19]. BioMed Central Ltd. Available from: https://doi.org/10.1186/s40248-019-0172-9.

13. Goldstein CA, Smith YR. Sleep, Circadian Rhythms, and Fertility [Internet]. Current Sleep Med Rep. 2016;2:206–17. Springer International Publishing.

[cited 2020 Sep 19]. Available from: https://link.springer.com/article/10.1007/s40675-016-0057-9.

14. Hirotsu C, Tufik S, Andersen ML. Sleep apnea as a potential threat to reproduction [Internet]. Sleep. 2014;37:1731–2. Associated Professional Sleep Societies, LLC. [cited 2020 Sep 19]. Available from: https://www.ncbi.nlm.nih.gov/pmc/articles/PMC4196055/.

15. Kim S, Cho K-S. Obstructive sleep apnea and testosterone deficiency. 2018

16. Seet E, Chung F. Obstructive sleep apnea: preoperative assessment [Internet]. Anesthesiol Clin. 2010;28:199–215. [cited 2020 Oct 4]. Available from: https://pubmed.ncbi.nlm.nih.gov/20488390/.

Sleep-disordered breathing results from either a static or a dynamic airway obstruction. A static obstruction could be due to either a structural abnormality in the upper airway or a space occupying lesion causing an airway obstruction.

The aim of this chapter is to understand the anatomical aspects, so as to be able to relate to them in the context of upper airway surgery for sleep apnea.

4.1   Anatomy of Nasal Airway

The upper airway begins from the nasal vestibule and ends at the larynx. The nasal cavity is wider below than above, and widest and vertically deepest in its central region. It communicates with the frontal, ethmoidal, maxillary, and sphenoidal paranasal sinuses.

The areas of importance in the nasal airway for an understanding of OSA are:

– Nasal valve
– Medial wall/septum
– Lateral wall of the nose
– Nasal mucosa

Nasal Valve It is composed of an external and an internal component.

The external nasal valve is bound laterally by the nasal alae and bony pyriform aperture, medially by the columella, and inferiorly by the nasal floor [1].

The internal nasal valve is the NARROWEST region of the nasal cavity and is bound by the cartilaginous portion of septum medially, lower border of the upper lateral cartilage superiorly, and head of the inferior turbinate anteriorly. The angle formed at the internal nasal valve is 10–15 degrees [1]. If there is narrowing at the level of the nasal valve, there is nasal obstruction, which leads to mouth breathing and sleep-disordered breathing (Fig. 4.1).

4.1.1   Medial Wall/Septum

The medial wall of the nasal cavity is the nasal septum formed primarily by the vomer and the perpendicular plate of the ethmoid in its bony part and septal cartilage in the cartilaginous part (Fig. 4.2).

A deviation of the nasal septum leads to nasal obstruction and is one of the most common causes for static obstruction in the upper airway.

4.1.2   Lateral Wall

The lateral wall of the nasal cavity contains three projections of variable sizes called the inferior, middle, and superior nasal conchae or turbinates. The nasal conchae or turbinates curve inferome-

Fig. 4.1 Anatomy of Internal nasal valve

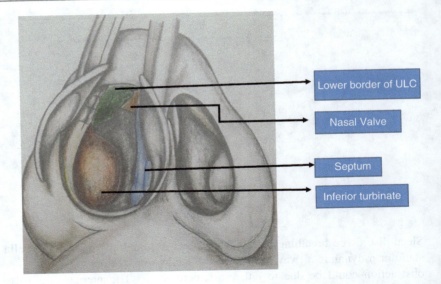

Lower border of ULC

Nasal Valve

Septum

Inferior turbinate

Fig. 4.2 Anatomy of septum

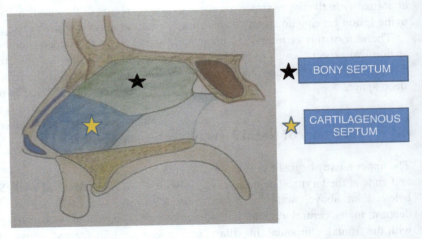

★ BONY SEPTUM

☆ CARTILAGENOUS SEPTUM

dially, each roofing a groove, or meatus, which open into the nasal cavity. There are three meatus in the nose, which are responsible for draining certain vital structures within them (Fig. 4.3).

– The anterior group of sinuses drains into the middle meatus of the nose and posterior ethmoids drain into the superior meatus and the sphenoid sinus drains into the sphenoethmoidal recess.
– Sinusitis and nasal polyposis are potential causes of SDB.
– Inferior turbinate hypertrophy may occur due to allergies or an imbalance between the sympathetic and the parasympathetic nervous system and this could be a cause of nasal obstruction and SDB.
– Concha Bullosa is an air filled pneumatization of the middle turbinate and this could lead to an obstruction of the airway.

4.2 Anatomy of the Pharyngeal Airway

4.2.1 Anatomy of the Nasopharynx

The nasopharynx is the part of the pharynx posterior to the nasal cavities and above the level of the junction of the hard and soft palate. The naso-

Fig. 4.3 Anatomy of Lateral wall

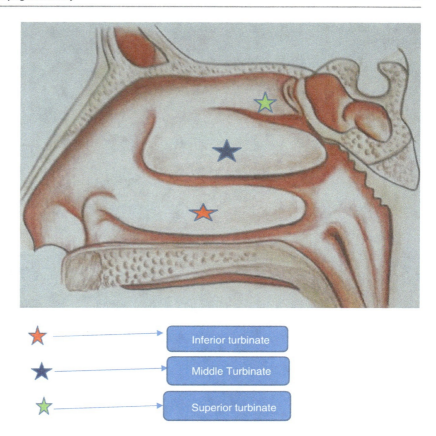

pharynx has a roof, floor, and walls on its posterior and lateral sides.

The roof and posterior wall merge smoothly and are formed by the mucoperiosteum which lies on the body of the sphenoid, the basisphenoid, and the basiocciput.

The floor of the nasopharynx is formed anteriorly by the superior surface of the soft palate which is continuous with the floor of the nasal cavities. Posteriorly, the floor is deficient where the nasopharynx communicates inferiorly with the oropharynx through the pharyngeal isthmus. The main feature of the lateral wall is the opening of the Eustachian tube. This is covered by a tubal elevation called torus tubarius.

Posterior to the tubal elevation is the lateral pharyngeal recess (fossa of Rosenmuller).

The pharyngeal opening of the auditory tube (pharyngotympanic tube ostium, Eustachian tube opening, or orifice) is approximately 1 cm behind the posterior end of the inferior turbinate.

The salpingopharyngeal mucosal fold extends inferiorly from the posterior part of the tubal elevation and is raised by the salpingopharyngeus muscle.

The salpingopalatine mucosal fold extends anteriorly from the anterior part of the tubal elevation to the superior surface of the palate.

4.2.2 Applied Aspects

– Adenoids, which are the lymphoid tissue of the nasopharynx, are often sites of obstruction in pediatric OSA.
– A prominent salpingopharyngeal fold causes a lateral collapse of the nasopharynx and thus obstructs the nasopharynx (Fig. 4.4).

Fig. 4.4 Anatomy of Nasopharynx

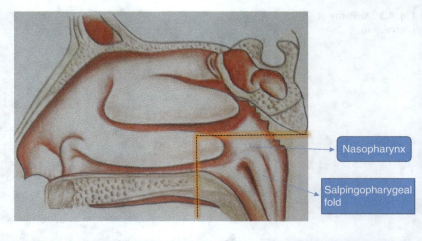

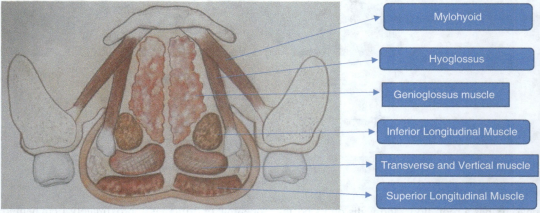

Fig. 4.5 Anatomy of Tongue (Axial)

4.2.3   Anatomy of Oral Airway

The oral cavity extends from the lips anteriorly to the uvula and posteriorly to the anterior pillars. Laterally it is bound by the buccal mucosa, and superiorly the palate separates the nasal cavity from the oral cavity. Floor of mouth is related to the anterior two thirds of the tongue.

Tongue It is divided into two thirds anteriorly and one third posteriorly by the sulcus terminalis. This is a V shaped groove behind the circumvallate papillae.

The tongue consists of intrinsic and extrinsic muscles. The intrinsic muscles are superior and inferior longitudinal muscles, transverse and vertical muscles. The extrinsic muscles of the tongue are genioglossus, hyoglossus, styloglossus, and palatoglossus (Fig. 4.5).

The key muscle responsible for keeping the retroglossal airway patent is the genioglossus. The mechanoreceptors control the activity of genioglossus and are critical in maintaining upper airway patency in patients with SDB.

The hypoglossus is responsible for the depression and retraction of the tongue. Surgical

Fig. 4.6 Anatomy of tongue (Sagittal)

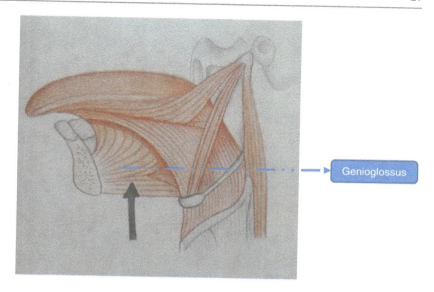

Genioglossus

advancement of this muscle is done to open the posterior airway space (Fig. 4.6).

4.2.4 Base of Tongue

The tongue is divided into two thirds anteriorly and one third posteriorly by the sulcus terminalis which lies behind the circumvallate papillae.

The hypertrophy of the tongue causes reduction in the retroglossal space, and this could be either due to lymphoid hypertrophy or muscular hypertrophy of the base of the tongue.

The lingual vessels are present in the base of tongue and the location of these vessels has to be confirmed preoperatively by an ultrasound examination to prevent bleeding while reducing the base of tongue (Fig. 4.7).

4.2.5 Anatomy of Oropharynx

4.2.5.1 Soft Palate

The soft palate is a mobile flexible partition forming the floor of the nasopharynx and the roof of the oropharynx anteriorly. Its movement is controlled by two groups of muscular sphincters which pull the palate up and back to close the nasopharynx and down and forward to close the oropharyngeal isthmus.

The soft palate is formed by the expanded tendons of the tensor palatini muscles which join in a median raphe called the palatine aponeurosis.

The aponeurosis is attached to the posterior edge of the hard palate and to its inferior surface behind the palatine crest.

Near the midline, it splits to enclose the uvular muscle and all the other muscles of the soft palate are attached to it. A fibrous aponeurosis occupies the anterior third of the velum. It is attached to the posterior edge of the hard palate and is continuous with the tendon of tensor veli palatini. The tensor tendon winds around the hamulus to which it is partly attached and ascends to its origin in the scaphoid fossa, spine of the sphenoid bone, and membranous portion of the tympanic tube. It is this latter attachment which suggests that the tensor's primary function is related to Eustachian tube function rather than velar function (Fig. 4.8).

The primary velar muscles are the levator palatini, palatopharyngeal, and palatoglossus.

The levator palatini muscle which originates from the medial part of the Eustachian tube is the prime elevator of the velum.

The palatoglossus and palatopharyngeus arise from the back of the palatal aponeurosis and maxillary tuberosity. The palatoglossus is a thin sheet of muscle that extends to form the anterior pillar of the fauces.

Fig. 4.7 Anatomy of base of tongue

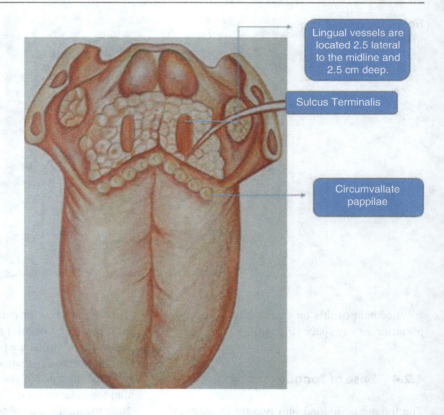

Lingual vessels are located 2.5 lateral to the midline and 2.5 cm deep.

Sulcus Terminalis

Circumvallate pappilae

Fig. 4.8 Palatal Aponeurosis

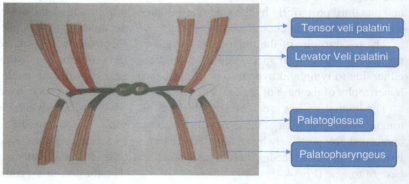

Tensor veli palatini

Levator Veli palatini

Palatoglossus

Palatopharyngeus

The palatopharyngeus is a much more substantial muscle that is split into two heads by the insertion of the levator palatini and which runs down to form the posterior pillar of fauces and inserts into the thyroid cartilage and pharyngeal aponeurosis (Fig. 4.9).

The diagram represents the slings of three muscles and their intersection when inserted into the palate (Fig. 4.10).

The palatopharyngeus and palatoglossus act as depressors and all three muscles act to lengthen the velum. The last muscle to consider is the muscularis uvulae, which runs anteroposteriorly from the posterior nasal spine to the uvula beneath the nasal mucosa.

4.2.5.2 Applied Aspects

The collapsible segment posterior to the soft palate is called the RETROPALATAL space and the space below that, behind the base of tongue is called the RETROGLOSSAL SPACE.

Any compromise in this space is one of the most important aspects in adult OSA.

Fig. 4.9 Muscular Anatomy of palate

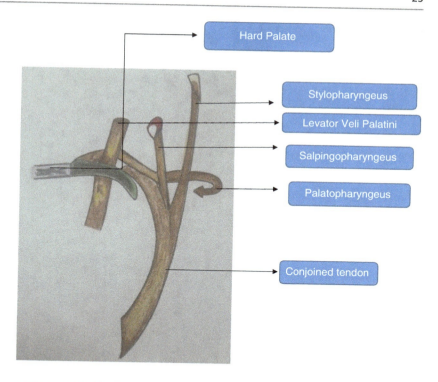

Fig. 4.10 Anatomy of Sling Muscles of palate

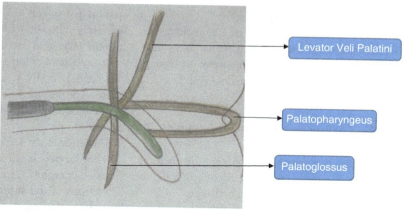

4.2.5.3 Oropharynx

The oropharynx extends from the junction of the hard and soft palates to the level of the floor of the vallecula. Anteriorly, it starts at the palatoglossal folds (anterior faucial pillar) formed by the underlying palatoglossus muscle passing from the undersurface of the palate to the side of the tongue. Just posterior to this, the palatopharyngeal fold (posterior faucial pillar) passes of the soft palate to

the side wall of the pharynx where it fades away. Beneath this is the palatopharyngeus muscle.

In the space between the two folds lie the palatine tonsils.

The superior wall is formed by the inferior surface of the soft palate and uvula. Below the oropharyngeal isthmus—the anterior wall is formed by the tongue base, behind the vallate papillae, and below this are the valleculae.

Fig. 4.11 Anatomy of Pharynx

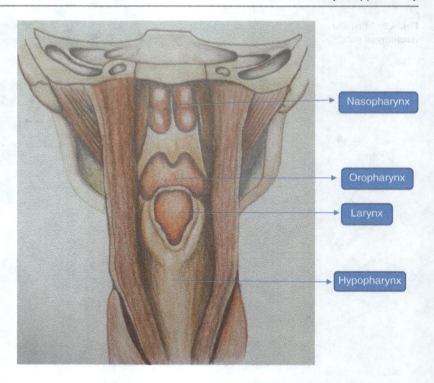

Nasopharynx

Oropharynx

Larynx

Hypopharynx

4.2.5.4 Palatine Tonsil

The palatine tonsil is a mass of lymphoid tissue situated in the lateral wall of the oropharynx, where it lies within the tonsillar fossa between the diverging palatopharyngeal and palatoglossal arches.

4.2.6 Larynx and Laryngopharynx

The laryngopharynx or hypopharynx lies behind the larynx. It extends from the tip of epiglottis to the lower border of the cricoid cartilage.

The segment capable of collapsing here is the retroepiglottic space.

The dimensions of this retroepiglottic space can be increased by pulling the hyoid bone anteriorly by a surgical intervention (Fig. 4.11).

4.2.7 Larynx

The larynx is located in the anterior compartment of the neck, suspended from the hyoid bone, and spanning between C3 and C6. It is continuous inferiorly with the trachea, and opens superiorly into the laryngeal part of the pharynx.

It is covered anteriorly by the infrahyoid muscles, and laterally by the lobes of the thyroid gland. The larynx is also closely related to the major blood vessels of the neck, which ascend laterally to it.

Posterior to the larynx is the esophagus.

The larynx is divided into three subdivisions—supraglottis, glottis, and subglottis.

Lesions of the supraglottis could obstruct the laryngeal inlet and thus the airway.

Primary epiglottic collapse is a condition where the epiglottis is lax and floppy causing airway obstruction while breathing.

Laryngeal webs at the level of the vocal cords or bilateral abductor paralysis causes the vocal cords to be in midline and paramedian position occluding the airway and these patients are most often non-compliant to PAP therapy (Fig. 4.12).

Fig. 4.12 Upper airway anatomy

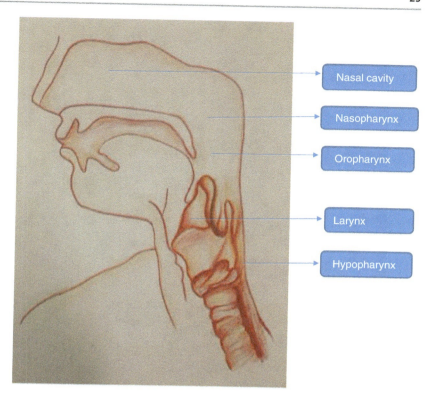

Nasal cavity

Nasopharynx

Oropharynx

Larynx

Hypopharynx

Reference

1. Dalgorf DM, Harvey RJ. Anatomy of the nose and paranasal sinuses. In: Scott-Brown's otorhinolaryngology head and neck surgery [Internet]. 8th ed. Boca Raton: CRC Press; 2019. p. 961–76. [cited 2021 Mar 14]. Available from: https://www.taylorfrancis.com/chapters/anatomy-nose-paranasal-sinuses-dustin-dalgorf-richard-harvey/e/10.1201/9780203731031-88.

Upper Airway Resistance Syndrome

5

Upper airway resistance syndrome (UARS) was first described in pediatric patients in 1982. Around a decade later, Guilleminault et al. first used the term UARS to describe the syndrome in adults in 1993 [1].

5.1 Definition

UARS is defined by the occurrence of excessive daytime sleepiness unexplained by any cause and associated with more than 50% of respiratory events that are non-apneic and non-hypopneic (i.e., RERAs). RERAs are characterized by a progressive increase in respiratory effort [2] (Table 5.1).

5.2 Pathophysiology

Abnormal inspiratory and expiratory flow dynamics results in increased airway collapsibility. Preserved upper airway reflexes in UARS lead to intermediate collapsibility resulting in an abnormal respiratory effort associated with increased airway resistance without significant oxygen desaturation. This in turn results in increased vagal tone which is responsible for hypotension, lower heart rate, and orthostatic symptoms during sleep and occasionally during wakefulness. On termination of the respiratory event, the vagal tone decreases resulting in increased heart rate. Persistent sensory input is also responsible for frequent arousals in

Table 5.1 UARS Definitions

Upper Airway Resistance Syndrome Definitions			
Authors	Clinical Criteria	Polysomnographic criteria	
Kristo et al., (2005)	EDS (ESS > 10)	Pes ≤12cmH2O	AHI < 5/hour., arousal index ≥10/hour, RERA ≥5/hour
Guilleminault et al.	EDS or fatigue	Pes and flow limitation by nasal cannula	AHI < 5, RDI > 5 per Hour, oxygen saturation > 92%
Loube et al., (2009)	EDS	Inductance plethysmography pes ≤ 12 cm H2O	AHI < 5 per hour, RERA > 10 per hour
Stoohs et al., (2009)	EDS or fatigue	Flow limitation by nasal cannula	AHI < 5 per hour, presence of RERA
Pépinetal., (2012)	EDS	Pes, flow limitation by nasal cannula	RERA as more than 50% of respiratory events

EDS Excessive Daytime Sleepiness, *ESS* Epworth Sleepiness Scale, *Pes* Esophageal pressure, *AHI* Apnea/Hypopnea Index, *RERA* Respiratory Event-Related Arousal, *RDI* Respiratory Disturbance Index

© The Author(s), under exclusive license to Springer Nature Singapore Pte Ltd. 2022
D. S. Deenadayal, V. Bommakanti, *Management of Snoring and Obstructive Sleep Apnea*,
https://doi.org/10.1007/978-981-16-6620-9_5

Table 5.2 Differences in pathophysiology of OSA and UARS

Differences in Pathophysiology of OSA and UARS	
Obstructive Sleep Apnea	Upper Airway Resistance Syndrome
Upper airway reflexes blunted	Upper airway reflexes preserved
Apneas and hypopneas are main respiratory events	Respiratory effort-related arousals are the main respiratory events
Upper airway collapsibility is more	Upper airway collapsibility is intermediate
Oxygen desaturation <92%	Oxygen desaturation >92%
Increased sympathetic tone during sleep	Increased vagal tone during sleep

Table 5.3 Clinical Features associated with UARS

Clinical Features Associated with UARS	
Daytime symptoms	Excessive daytime sleepiness fatigue Morning headaches Myalgias Difficulty in concentrating
Sleep disturbances	Frequent nocturnal awakenings difficulties initiating sleep insomnia Bruxism Restless leg syndrome unrefreshing sleep
Autonomic nervous system	Hypotension Orthostasis Cold hands and feet
Functional somatic syndrome associations	Depression anxiety Chronic fatigue syndrome Irritable bowel syndrome fibromyalgia
Polysomnographic abnormalities	Increased RERAs Increase nocturnal arousals increased CAP rate Alpha intrusion during sleep

UARS. This is in contrast to OSA wherein upper airway reflexes are blunted and hypoxia results in sympathetic hyperactivity and arousals [3] (Table 5.2).

5.3 Clinical Features

- UARS patients are significantly younger and less overweight with equal incidence in both males and females.
- Patients with UARS typically complain of excessive daytime, sleepiness, fatigue, difficulty concentrating, morning headaches, unrefreshing sleep, frequent nocturnal awakening and tend to have more difficulty falling back to sleep.
- Individuals most likely affected are those with abnormal airway anatomy, including decreased retrolingual space, narrow nasal passages, or a small neck circumference.
- Patients exhibit the classical long face syndrome with a short and narrow chin and reduced mouth opening. There is classically a "click" and a subluxation when opening the temporomandibular articulation, which may be evidenced by palpation [2].
- Patients may have symptoms of abnormal autonomic function, including lightheadedness or dizziness upon rising from a supine or sitting position, cold hands and feet, and low resting blood pressures (defined as a systolic blood pressure of <105 mmHg with a diastolic blood pressure of <65 mmHg).
- Other presentations include parasomnias with sleepwalking and sleep terrors, myalgia, gastroesophageal reflux, depression, and anxiety, in addition to functional somatic syndromes such as headaches, sleep onset insomnia, and irritable bowel syndrome. Therefore, UARS can commonly be misdiagnosed as chronic fatigue syndrome, fibromyalgia, or psychiatric disorders such as ADD/ADHD or depressive disorders [4] (Tables 5.3 and 5.4).

5.4 Diagnosis

Diagnosis of UARS can be diagnosed with symptoms of excessive daytime somnolence and polysomnography showing more than 10 EEG arousal per hour associated with increased intrathoracic pressure [5].

1. Polysomnography–.
   - Apnea–hypopnea index is less than 5.
   - The oxygen saturation is usually>92%.
   - Increased frequency of respiratory effort-related arousals (RERAs; RERA index>5 h-1).

Table 5.4 Differences between OSA and UARS

Differences in clinical features in upper airway resistance syndrome (UARS) and obstructive sleep apnea–hypopnea syndrome (OSAHS)

Features	UARS	OSAHS
Age	All ages	Children Male >40 year old female after menopause
Male: Female ratio	1:1	2:1
Sleep onset	Insomnia	Fast
Snoring	Common	Almost always
Apnea	No	Common
Daytime symptoms	Tiredness Fatigue	Sleepiness (less common in children
Body habitus	Slim or normal	Obese
Somatic functional complaints	Fibromyalgia, chronic pains, headaches	Rare
Orthostatic symptoms	Cold hands/feet, fainting, dizziness	Rare
Blood pressure	Low or normal	High
Neck circumference	Normal	Large

- Flow limitation is commonly present, identified as an abnormal contour in the nasal pressure transducer signal waveform.
2. Esophageal Manometry (Pes).
   - Gold standard.
   - A characteristic finding is a Pes crescendo defined as a progressive increase in negative peak inspiratory pressure with each breath that terminates with an electroencephalogram (EEG) arousal [3].
   - Other changes include "sustained continuous respiratory effort"; the Pes tracing shows a stable and persistently abnormal negative peak inspiratory pressure, different from the baseline pressure and present for more than four breaths, often for longer than 1 min [3].
   - The termination of both events is called Pes reversal, defined as a decrease in respiratory effort evident by a less negative peak inspiratory pressure, often without an associated EEG arousal [3].
3. Electroencephalogram (EEG).
   - Increased amounts of alpha frequency on EEG.
   - UARS patients have more theta and low alpha powers (7–9 Hz) during NREM sleep and more delta power during REM sleep [4].
   - Increase in delta frequency activity before Pes reversal along with increases in other frequencies following the event suggests that significant EEG changes occur with Pes events without a visible EEG arousal.
   - Cyclical alternating pattern (CAP) on EEG is another diagnostic feature. CAPs are a well-described pattern of non-REM sleep, defined as periodically occurring electrocortical events distinct from background EEG activity [3].
   - An increase in CAP frequency indicates sleep instability and/or disturbance in addition to central nervous system hyperactivity. CAP rate has been correlated with daytime symptoms of sleepiness and fatigue [3] (Table 5.5).

Table 5.5 Polysomnography and EEG in UARS and OSA

Polysomnography and EEG activity in UARS and OSAHS

Features	UARS	OSAHS
Sleep onset latency	Long	Short
AHI	<5	≥5
Minimum oxygen saturation	>92%	Often <92%
Respiratory effort-related arousals	Predominant	Minimal
Cyclic alternating pattern (CAP)	Frequent	Less common
Power spectral EEG analysis	Higher alpha wave power Higher delta waves in REM	Less alpha or delta waves

5.5   Treatment

Optimal treatment of UARS remains unknown.

CPAP THERAPY: CPAP therapy is the first line of treatment. CPAP treatment decreases transient arousals, increases percentage of NREM stages 3 and 4 and the sleep latency at MSLT [6]. Subjective daytime sleepiness, fatigue, and snoring also can improve after CPAP treatment.

ORAL APPLIANCES: Patients with UARS present a narrow posterior airway space behind the base of the tongue. Oral devices move the mandible and tongue forward in order to increase the oropharyngeal airway [7].

SURGICAL MANAGEMENT: Surgery may be considered in patients non-compliant/intolerant to CPAP therapy or in whom CPAP therapy has not shown much benefit. UARS may be associated with craniofacial anomalies that increase the upper airway resistance. Nasal obstruction can cause flow limitation and can lead to occlusion of the pharyngeal air way. Dental malocclusion, high arched palate, and narrow posterior airway space are also common findings. Surgical treatment of UARS consists of approaching the causes of the upper airway anatomical problems such as treatment of nasal allergies, nasal surgeries (septoplasty, turbinate reduction), palatal soft-tissue surgeries (Uvulopharyngoplasty, radiofrequency ablation of soft palate, etc.), genioglossus advancement, orthognathic surgery (maxillary mandibular advancement) [7].

References

1. Guilleminault C, Takaoka S. Signs and symptoms of obstructive sleep apnea and upper airway resistance syndrome. In: Sleep apnea and snoring. Philadelphia: Elsevier; 2009. p. 3–10.
2. Pépin JL, Guillot M, Tamisier R, Lévy P. The upper airway resistance Syndrome. Theatr Res Int. 2012 Jun;83(6):559–66. [cited 2020 Sep 28]. Available from: https://www.karger.com/Article/FullText/335839.
3. Masri TJ, Guilleminault C. Upper airway resistance syndrome [Internet]. Encyclopedia of sleep. Amsterdam: Elsevier; 2013. p. 269–274. Available from: https://doi.org/10.1016/B978-0-12-378610-4.00320-X.
4. Bao G, Guilleminault C. Upper airway resistance syndrome-one decade later. Curr Opin Pulm Med. 2004;10(6):461–7.
5. Upper Airway Resistance Syndrome – an overview | ScienceDirect Topics [Internet]. [cited 2021 Jul 5]. Available from: https://www.sciencedirect.com/topics/agricultural-and-biological-sciences/upper-airway-resistance-syndrome.
6. de Godoy LBM, Palombini LO, Guilleminaulth C, Poyares D, Tufik S, Togeiro SM. Treatment of upper airway resistance syndrome in adults: where do we stand? Sleep Sci [Internet]. 2015;8(1):42–8. Available from: https://doi.org/10.1016/j.slsci.2015.03.001
7. de Godoy LBM, Palombini LO, Guilleminaulth C, Poyares D, Tufik S, Togeiro SM. Treatment of upper airway resistance syndrome in adults: where do we stand? [Internet]. Sleep Science. 2015;8:42–8. FLASS. [cited 2021 Feb 22]. Available from: https://www.ncbi.nlm.nih.gov/pmc/articles/PMC4608900/.

History, Clinical Examination, and Diagnosis of Snoring and Obstructive Sleep Apnea–Hypopnea Syndrome

6

The first step in the management is to recognize the presence or absence of obstructive sleep apnea [OSA]. If present, the next step would be to recognize the severity. The diagnosis of this condition begins with a sleep-oriented history, physical examination, and the findings collected from an overnight sleep study.

6.1 History

Questions to be asked include those regarding a history of snoring or daytime sleepiness, any witnessed apneas by bed partner, choking or gasping episodes, morning headaches and dry throat, decreased concentration at work, memory loss, and decreased libido and irritability.

Additionally, an associated history of hypertension, diabetes, cardiac or cerebral diseases, chronic obstructive pulmonary disease, or depression should be collected.

There are many available questionnaires in literature to grade the severity of OSA. The most commonly used ones are

1. Epworth sleepiness score [1] (Table 6.1).
2. Stop Bang Questionnaire [2] (Table 6.2).
3. Stanford questionnaire [3] (Table 6.3).
4. Berlin questionnaire: [4] (Table 6.4).

A positive history, on screening, should mandate a comprehensive physical examination and a local examination. This will help the clinician in determining which diagnostics tests should be ordered and which co-morbidities must be managed, ultimately determining the treatment method that must be employed.

Table 6.1 Epworth Sleepiness Score (ESS)

Epworth Sleepiness Scale	
No chance of dozing =0 Slight chance of dozing = 1 Moderate chance of dozing = 2 High chance of dozing = 3	
Situation	Chance of Dozing
Sitting and reading	
Watching TV	
Sitting inactive in a public place (e.g., a theater or a meeting)	
As a passenger in a car for an hour without a break	
Lying down to rest in the afternoon when circumstances permit	
Sitting and talking to someone	
Sitting quietly after lunch without alcohol	
In a car stopped for a few minutes in traffic	
Total Score =	
Interpretation 0–7: It is unlikely that you are abnormally sleepy 8–9: You have an average amount of daytime sleepiness 10–11: You may be excessively sleepy depending upon the situation. You may want to consider seeking medical attention 16–24: You are excessively sleepy and should consider seeking medical attention	

Table 6.2 Stop Bang Questionnaire

Stop – Bang Questionnaire		
Snoring—Do you snore loudly (Loud enough to be heard through closed doors or your bed partner elbows you for snoring at night?)	Yes	No
Tired—Do you often feel tired, fatigued, or sleepy during the daytime? (such as falling asleep during driving)	Yes	No
Observed—Has anyone observed you stop breathing or choking/gasping during sleep?	Yes	No
Pressure—Do you have or are being treated for high blood pressure?	Yes	No
Body Mass Index—BMI > 35 kg/m^2?	Yes	No
Age—Older than 50 years?	Yes	No
Neck Circumference—For males ≥17 inches and for females ≥ inches (measured at level of Adam's apple)	Yes	No
Gender—Male?	Yes	No
Interpretation		
Low risk of OSA	Yes to 0–2 questions	
Intermediate risk of OSA	Yes to 3–4 questions	
High risk of OSA	Yes to 5–8 questions; Yes to 2 of 4 STOP questions + Gender is male; Yes to 2 of 4 STOP questions + BMI > 35 kg/m^2; Yes to 2 of 4 STOP questions + Neck circumference ≥ 17 inches (in male) or ≥ 16 inches (in female)	

Table 6.3 Stanford Questionnaire

Stanford Sleepiness Scale	
Indicate current level of sleepiness	
Degree of sleepiness	**Scale rating**
Feeling active and vital; alert; wide awake	1
Functioning at a high level, but not at peak; able to concentrate	2
Relaxed; awake; not at full alertness; responsive	3
A little foggy; not at peak; let down	4
Fogginess; beginning to lose interest in remaining awake; slowed down	5
Sleepiness; prefer to be lying down; fighting sleep; woozy	6
No longer fighting sleep; sleep onset soon; lost struggle to remain awake, having dream like thoughts	7
Asleep	X

6.2   Anthropometric Measurements in Suspected Patients of OSA

Body mass index: is calculated by the formula BMI = weight [Kg]/height [m]2 (Table 6.5).

In addition to the Body mass index, neck circumference and waist circumference are significant risk factors for predictors of OSA.

6.2.1   Neck Circumference

Neck circumference is measured at the level of the superior border of the cricothyroid membrane. This measurement is performed with the patient in an upright position.

A neck circumference of >40 cm [16 inches] in females and > 43 cm [17 inches] in males is a positive predictor for the presence of obstructive sleep apnea.

Patients with neck circumference more than 48 cm [19.2 inches] have a 20 fold increased risk of OSA [5].

6.2.2   Waist Circumference

Waist circumference is measured at the midpoint between the lower border of the rib cage and the

Table 6.4 Berlin Questionnaire

BERLIN QUESTIONAIRRE		
CATEGORY 1		
Do you snore?	☐ Yes ☐ No ☐ Don't know	
Your snoring is?	☐ Slightly louder than breathing ☐ As loud as talking ☐ Louder than talking ☐ Can be heard in adjacent room	
Describe your snoring frequency?	☐ Nearly everyday ☐ 3-4 times a week ☐ 1-2 times a week ☐ 1-2 times a month ☐ Never or nearly never	
Has your snoring ever bothered other people?	☐ Yes ☐ No	
Has anyone noticed that you quit breathing during your sleep?	☐ Nearly everyday ☐ 3-4 times a week ☐ 1-2 times a week ☐ 1-2 times a month ☐ Never or nearly never	
CATEGORY 2		
How often do you feel tired or fatigued after you sleep?	☐ Nearly everyday ☐ 3-4 times a week ☐ 1-2 times a week ☐ 1-2 times a month ☐ Never or nearly never	
During your wake time, do you feel tired, fatigued or not upto mark?	☐ Nearly everyday ☐ 3-4 times a week ☐ 1-2 times a week ☐ 1-2 times a month ☐ Never or nearly never	
Have you ever nodded off or fallen asleep while driving a vehicle?	☐ Yes ☐ No	
If yes, how often does it occur?	☐ Nearly everyday ☐ 3-4 times a week ☐ 1-2 times a week ☐ 1-2 times a month ☐ Never or nearly never	
CATEGORY 3		
Do you have high blood pressure	☐ Yes ☐ No	
Body Mass Index (kg/m²)		
INTERPRETATION		
☐ Category 1 Positive (≥2) ☐ Category 2 Positive (≥2) ☐ Category 3 Positive (1 or BMI > 30 kg/m²)		

iliac crest with the patient in an upright position. Central obesity has been positively associated with the occurrence of OSA [6].

Generally, abdominal obesity is defined as a WC of 90 cm or more in men or 80 cm or more in women in the Asian population and 94 cm or more in men or 80 cm or more in women in the Middle Eastern and Caucasian population [7].

Table 6.5 Body Mass Index

Body Mass Index	
18.5 kg/m² or less	Underweight
18.5 kg/m² to 24.9 kg/m²	Normal
25 kg/m² to 29.9 kg/m²	Overweight
30 kg/m² to 34.9 kg/m²	Obese
35 kg/m² to 39.9 kg/m²	Obese
40 kg/m² or greater	Extremely Obese

6.2.3 Craniofacial Factors

Craniofacial malformations have known to be associated with obstructive sleep apnea [8]. Clinicians check for the presence of mandibular retrognathia, micrognathia, macroglossia, and hypoplastic maxilla. These factors cause reduced retronasal, retroglossal, and retropalatal space.

6.3 Clinical Examination

6.3.1 Examination of Nose and Nasopharynx

Anterior rhinoscopy along with 0 degree rigid nasal endoscopy is performed to identify the presence of a deviated nasal septum or hypertrophic turbinate or nasal polyposis or any other mass occupying the nasal cavity which could be the cause of snoring and obstructive sleep apnea.

Also the nasopharynx is examined for any mass like adenoid, prominent salpingopharyngeal fold.

6.3.2 Examination of Oropharynx

The intent of examining the oropharynx is to check for the presence of any oropharyngeal narrowing. The classification that is widely used is the Friedman's classification. A revision of this classification was done by Friedman et al. in 2017 which is mentioned below [9]. This classification identifies the prognostic indicators for successful surgery for the treatment of obstructive sleep apnea. This grading is based on the tongue in its natural position inside the mouth. The position of the palate and the tonsils are assessed.

Friedman Tongue position: [9] (Figs. 6.1 and 6.2).

Tonsil grading: [9] (Figs. 6.3 and 6.4).

Staging: [9] (Table 6.6).

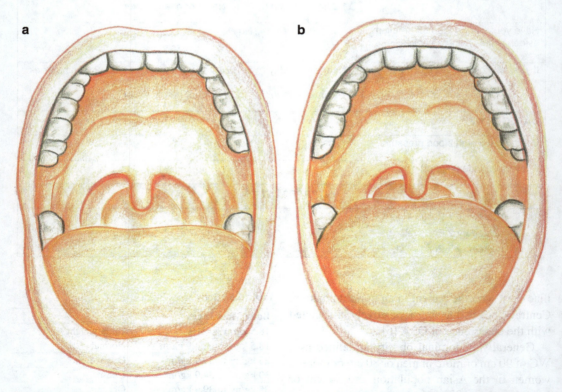

a   b

Fig. 6.1 (**a**) FTP I visualizes uvula and tonsil/pillars; (**b**) FTP IIa visualizes most of uvula but not the tonsil/pillars

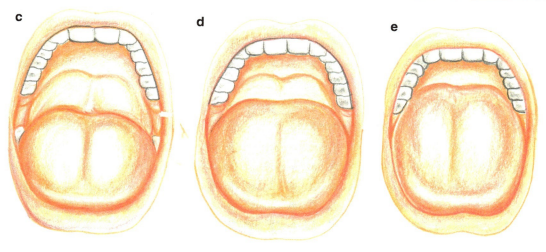

Fig. 6.2 (**c**) FTP IIb visualizes entire soft palate to the uvular base; (**d**) FTP III shows some of the soft palate with the distal end absent; (**e**) FTP IV visualizes only the hard palate

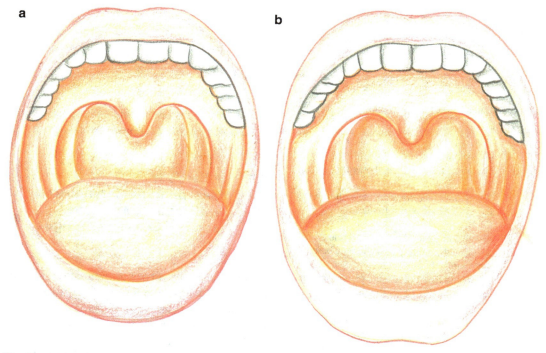

Fig. 6.3 (**a**) Size 0: Absence of tonsillar tissue; (**b**) Size 1: Within the pillars

It is important to assess the tongue base if there is a lingual tonsil hypertrophy or there is a muscular tongue base.

Lingual tonsil hypertrophy is classified as [9] (Table 6.7, Figs. 6.5, 6.6, 6.7, 6.8, and 6.9).

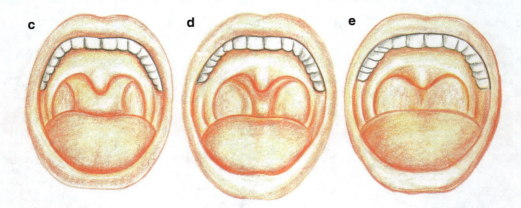

Fig. 6.4 (**c**) Size 2: Extended to the pillars; (**d**) Size 3: Extended past the pillars; (**e**) Size 4: Extended to the midline

Table 6.6 Friedman Staging System

Friedman Staging System as Determined by Friedman Tongue Position (FTP), Tonsil Size, and BMI			
Stage	FTP	Tonsil Size	BMI
I	I, IIa, IIb	3 or 4	<40
II	I, IIa, IIb	0, 1, or 2	<40
	III or IV	3 or 4	<40
III	III or IV	0, 1, or 2	<40
IV[a]	I – IV	0–4	>40

[a]All patients with significant craniofacial or other anatomic abnormalities

Table 6.7 Lingual Tonsil Hypertrophy

Lingual Tonsil Hypertrophy	
Grade 0	Complete absence of lymphoid tissue on the tongue base
Grade 1	Lymphoid tissue scattered over the tongue base
Grade 2	Lymphoid tissue covering the entirety of the tongue base with a limited vertical thickness
Grade 3	Significantly raised lymphoid tissue covering the entirety of the tongue base, approximately 5–10 mm in thickness
Grade 4	Lymphoid tissue of about 1 cm or more in thickness, rising above the tip of the epiglottis

The vertical depth of the lingual tonsils is a clinical approximation that should be judged by the otolaryngologist, with grade 3 being the first stage in which the tonsils have significant vertical height

6.4   OSA Scoring (Table 6.8)

6.4.1   Examination of Hypopharynx and Larynx

- An indirect laryngoscopic examination with an IDL mirror or now, most often, a 70 degree

videolaryngoscopy is performed to assess the pathology in the hypopharynx and larynx.

6.5   Fiberoptic Nasopharyngolaryngoscopy with Muller's Maneuver and End Expiratory Tongue Position

Fibreoptic upper airway examination is conducted to identify the levels of obstruction. In case of any obstruction in the area of the nose/nasopharynx/oropharynx/laryngopharynx, a Muller's maneuver, which is the forced voluntary inspiration with the mouth and nose closed, is performed. This helps to determine the level and degree of the obstruction present in these areas.

In the areas of the nasopharynx/oropharynx and at the tongue base, after performing the Muller's maneuver, any lateral, anteroposterior, or circumferential collapse is noted carefully.

Since this procedure is done in awake patients, the results may not be an accurate rep-

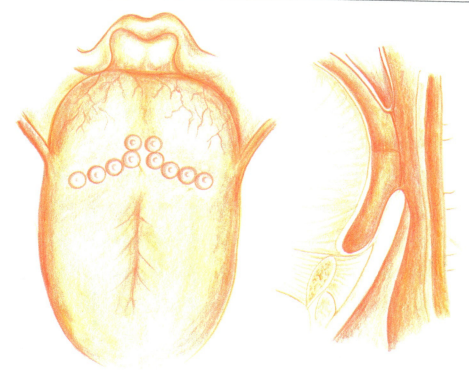

Fig. 6.5 Grade 0 Lingual Tonsil with complete absence of lymphoid tissue on tongue base

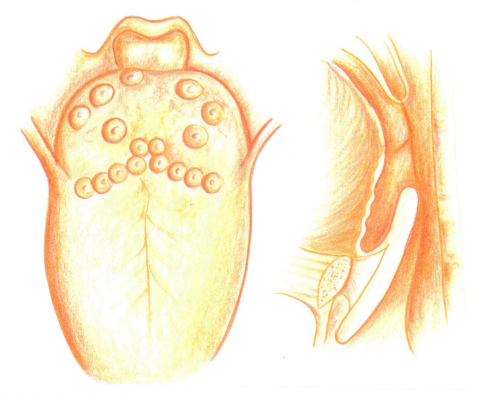

Fig. 6.6 Grade 1 Lingual Tonsil Hypertrophy with lymphoid tissue scattered over tongue base

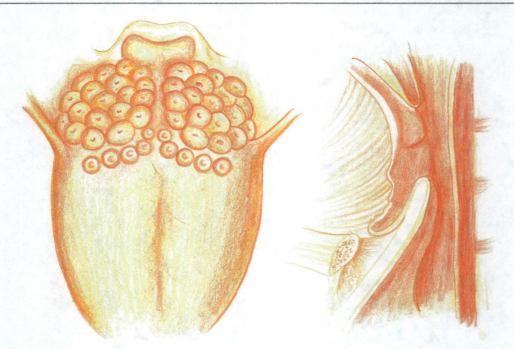

Fig. 6.7 Grade 2 Lingual Tonsil Hypertrophy with lymphoid tissue covering entire tongue base with limited vertical thickness

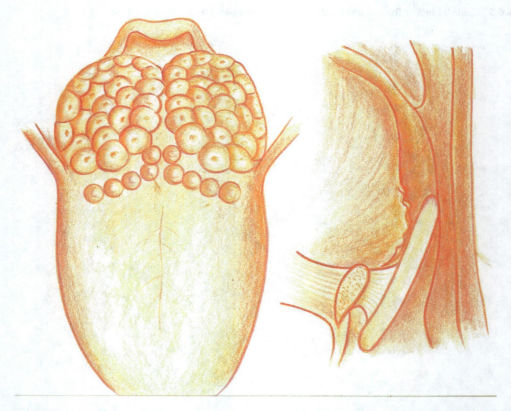

Fig. 6.8 Grade 3 Lingual Tonsil Hypertrophy with significantly raised lymphoid tissue covering the entirety of the tongue base, approximately 5–10 mm in thickness

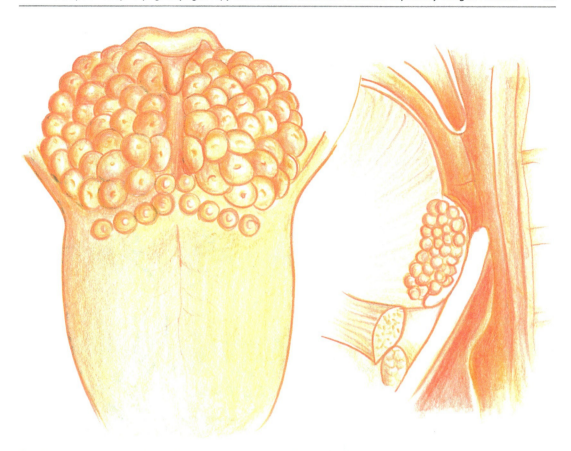

Fig. 6.9 Grade 4 Lingual Tonsil Hypertrophy with lymphoid tissue of about 1 cm or more in thickness, rising above the tip of the epiglottis

Table 6.8 OSA Scoring

Feature	Score
Friedman Tongue Position (FTP)	0–4
Tonsil grading	0–4
Body mass index (BMI)	0–4
BMI <20 = 0, BMI: 20–25 = 1, BMI: 25–30 = 2, BMI: 30–40 = 3, BMI >40 = 4	
Interpretation	
Any value greater than 8 is considered positive for OSA	
Any value less than 4 is considered negative for OSA	

resentation of the actual collapse which happens during sleep. But the results can be taken as representative.

6.5.1   Procedure

This procedure is done in an awake patient in a semi-upright position. The nasal cavity is anes-thetized by placing pledgets of cotton dipped in 4 percent xylocaine solution. A fiberoptic nasopha-ryngoscope is passed into the nasal cavity on both sides and any pathology of the nose, like a nasal valve narrowing/DNS/Turbinate hypertro-phy/Polyps, is identified.

The scope is now advanced from one side of the nasal cavity into the choanae and nasophar-ynx. Any pathology in this area, like choanal atresia/adenoid hypertrophy/prominent salpingo-pharyngeal folds/any space occupying lesions, is assessed. The Muller's maneuver is also per-formed here to check for any collapse, i.e. retro-palatal circumferential, lateral, or AP collapse.

6.5.2   Palatal Phenophype

The position of the junction of hard and soft pal-ate is important and the curvature at this junction is called as the genu or knee. It is very important to assess this for the surgical planning. Classically, three retropalatal vertical shape patterns are described [10] which are-

- A vertical soft palate is the one where the hard palate extends posteriorly with a sharper genu. Here the pharyngeal isthmus is narrow at both the velopharynx and the hard palate.
- An intermediate type in which the airway is open at the hard palate and narrow at the genu and velum.
- An oblique type where the pharyngeal isthmus is open at the hard palate and narrows at the velopharynx.

6.5.3   Modified Moores Tonguebase Classifcation

The original Moores classification categorized the lower pharyngeal obstruction based on lateral cephalometric radiographs, while the modified classification is based on endoscopic evaluation [11] (Tables 6.9 and 6.10).

The scope is then advanced from the nasopharynx to the velum which is the junction of the nasopharynx and oropharynx. The Muller's maneuver is performed here and the type of collapse, whether anteroposterior, circumferential, or lateral, is assessed.

The scope is then advanced further down to visualize the base of tongue. The patient is asked to take a deep breath and then exhale and then hold the breath in expiration for 10 seconds. At this end of this expiration, the position of tongue is visualized and the residual airway space at the base of tongue is assessed.

Any lymphoid hypertrophy or muscular hypertrophy at the base of the tongue is noted.

The scope is now advanced to visualize the larynx. The shape of the epiglottis, the supraglottis, and the vocal cords is noted. The movement of the vocal cords is assessed to check for bilateral abductor palsy of the cords (Table 6.11).

Isolated site of obstruction is found only in 15 percent of patients. In 85% of patients there are multiple sites of obstruction.

Table 6.9 Modified Moore's Tongue Base Classification

Modified Moore's Tongue Base Classification		
Type A	Only proximal (tongue base) obstruction	
Type B	Proximal (tongue base) and distal (epiglottic) obstruction	
Type C	Only distal (epiglottic) obstruction	

The sites of obstruction can be scored as follows:

0—No obstruction
1—Single site of obstruction.
2—Two levels.

Advantage: This procedure is easy to perform and it helps to assess the dynamic changes that occur in the airway. It is also cost effective.

Disadvantage: This technique has been criticized since it cannot show the different levels of obstruction at the same time. It is performed when the patient is awake in a semi-sitting position and every patient cannot create an optimal negative pressure.

Table 6.10 Patterns of upper pharyngeal airway collapse

Patterns of upper pharyngeal airway collapse			
Shape	Site of obstruction		Treatment
Oblique/funnel	Velum		Minimally invasive soft palate procedures
Intermediate	Velum and genu		Soft tissue palatal surgeries
Vertical/tubular	Velum, genu, and hard palate		Palatal advancement

Table 6.11 Classification of levels of obstruction

Classification of Levels of Obstruction	
Level 1	Nose and nasopharynx
Level 2	Velopharyngeal sphincter and oropharynx
Level 3	Base of tongue and superior hypopharynx
Level 4	Larynx and inferior hypopharynx

6.6 Polysomnography[PSG]

This test is considered as the "gold standard" for diagnosing SDB and other sleep disorders. As per the American Academy of Sleep Medicine standard of practice guidelines, there are four levels of sleep study [12].

- Level 1: Attended cardiorespiratory polysomnography with at least 7 signals.
- Level 2: Unattended, cardiorespiratory polysomnography at home with at least 7 signals.
- Level 3: Unattended portable sleep apnea testing with at least 4 signals including airflow, respiratory effort, oxygen saturation, ECG or heart rate or pulse rate.
- Level 4: Unattended one or two signal recordings such as actigraphy or oximetry.

According to AASM (American Academy of Sleep Medicine) standards, a full night PSG is routinely indicated for the diagnosis of SRBDs and for continuous positive airway pressure (CPAP) titration in patients with a documented diagnosis of a SRBD for whom PAP is warranted [12].

Because of the first-night effect, where the patient is not comfortable in doing a sleep study, it is considered ideal to perform a sleep study for 2 to 3 nights and then take an average [13].

For all patients of suspected OSA with co-morbidities, a level 1 and level 2 sleep study is advised [14].

For screening in general population, a level 3 study is indicated [14]. The level 4 study is often not indicated in the diagnosis of OSA [12].

6.6.1   Clinical Definitions

Obstructive Apnea: It is defined as the cessation of airflow for at least 10 seconds with an active effort to breath.

Central Apnea: It is defined as the cessation of airflow for at least 10 seconds when there is no effort to breath.

Mixed Apnea: It is defined as the cessation of airflow for at least 10 seconds. The event initially begins as a central apnea and progresses by the end to a point where is an effort to breath without airflow.

Hypopnea: It is defined as at least a 50% reduction in the airflow as compared to baseline lasting for at least 10 seconds or a 30% reduction in the thoracoabdominal movement or airflow as compared to baseline at least for 10 sec with $>/=4\%$ oxygen desaturation.

Respiratory Effort-Related Arousal (RERA): It is a sequence of breaths with increasing respiratory effort leading to arousal from sleep, as shown by progressively more negative esophageal pressure for at least 10 sec preceding an arousal with resumption of more normal pressures. They are increased in upper airway resistance syndrome.

Apnea Hypopnea Index (AHI): it is the total number of apneas and hypopneas per hour of sleep (Table 6.12).

Respiratory Distress Index (RDI): It is the average number of apneas, hypopneas, and breathing-related arousals per hour of sleep (Tables 6.13 and 6.14).

A typical level 3 home sleep study is reported as below.

Table 6.12 AHI in adults

Apnea Hypopnea Index in Adults	
Less than 5	Normal
5–15	Mild OSA
15–30	Moderate OSA
>30	Severe OSA

Table 6.13 Respiratory Distress Index

Respiratory Distress Index	
< 5 events per hour	No OSA
5–14.9 events per hour	Mild OSA
15–29.9 events per hour	Moderate OSA
>30 events per hour	Severe OSA

Table 6.14 Comparison between AHI, RERA and RDI

	AHI	RERA	RDI
Definition	Apneas + Hypopneas per hour of sleep	Increasing respiratory effort (and thus decreasing esophageal pressures) for 10 sec or more leading to an arousal from sleep, but one that does not fulfill the criteria for a hypopnea or apnea	AHI + RERA per hour of sleep
Diagnosis	Nasal/oral airflow, thoracoabdominal effort, oxygen saturations, EEG	Nasal/oral airflow, thoracoabdominal effort, esophageal manometry, oxygen saturations, EEG	–
OSA	Increased	Maybe increased	Increased
UARS	Normal	Increased	Increased

Patient data

First name:	
Last Name:	
Street:	
City, ST, Zip:	
Phone:	

Patient ID:	
DOB:	06-06-1985
Height:	170 cm
Weight:	83 kg
BMI:	28.7 kg/m²

Recording

Date:	18-09-2019
Start:	22:00 .
End:	5:55 .
Duration:	7 h 55 min

Evaluation

Start:	22:10 .
End:	5:52 .
Duration:	7 h 6 min

—— AHI* ——

Normal range | Suspected pathological breathing disorder

Result (25)

* See Clinical Guide for abbreviations and ResMed standard parameters

Analysis   (Flow evaluation period: 7 h 6 min / SpO2 evaluation period: 7 h 44 min)

Indices		Normal	Result	
AHI*:	25.2	< 5 / h	Average breaths per minute [bpm]:	12.86
RI*:	30.4	< 5	Breaths:	5476
Apnea index:	14.8	< 5 / h	Apneas:	105
UAI:	1.1		Unclassified apneas:	8 (8%)
OAI:	12.3		Obstructive apneas:	87 (83%)
CAI:	1.1		Central apneas:	8 (8%)
MAI:	0.3		Mixed apneas:	2 (2%)
Hypopnea index:	10.4	< 5 / h	Hypopneas:	74
% Flow lim. Br. without Sn (FL):	22	< Approx. 60	Flow lim. Br. without Sn (FL):	1198
% Flow lim. Br. with Sn (FS):	29	< Approx. 40	Flow lim. Br. with Sn (FS):	1567
			Snoring events:	4807
ODI Oxygen Desaturation Index*:	22.2	< 5 / h	No. of desaturations:	172
Average saturation:	94	94% - 98%	Saturation 90% :	55 min (12%)
Lowest desaturation:	71	-	Saturation 85% :	31 min (7%)
Lowest saturation:	71	90% - 98%	Saturation 80% :	8 min (2%)
Baseline Saturation:	97	%		
Minimum pulse:	40	> 40 bpm		
Maximum pulse:	92	< 90 bpm		
Average pulse:	56	bpm		
Proportion of probable CS epochs:	0	0%		

Analysis status: Analyzed automatically

Analysis parameters used (Default)

Apnea [20%; 10s; 80s; 1.0s; 20%; 60%; 8%]; Hypopnea [70%; 10s; 100s; 1.0s]; Snoring [6.0%; 0.3s; 3.5s; 0.5s]; Desaturation [4.0%]; CSR [0.50]

6.6.2 How to Report a Level 3 Sleep Study

The first part of report consists of patient data, anthropometric data, the time of recording, etc.

The second part of the report describes the AHI and the risk of OSA (Table 6.15).

The third part consists of the parameters measured in the test which includes the respiratory index, total number of apneas per hour, total number of hypopneas per hour, presence of any central apneas, total number of snoring events, flow limitations without snoring, and flow limitation with snoring.

Inspiratory flow limitation (IFL) can be observed as flattening of the flow tracing on PSG. Physiologically, IFL indicates absence of an increase in flow despite an elevation in negative intrathoracic pressure indicating increasing effort. Basically the importance of flow limitation lies in identifying other forms of sleep-disordered breathing like upper airway resistance syndrome. Flow limitation without snoring is an indicator of probable nasal obstruction and flow limitation with snoring is an indicator of palatal and tongue base obstruction [15, 16].

6.7 Drug Induced Sleep Endoscopy [DISE]

Due to the difficulty in establishing the site of obstruction in a conscious patient undergoing the diagnosis of OSAS, Croft and Pringle first proposed sleep endoscopy in 1991 [17]. They demonstrated the utility of passing a fiberoptic endoscope through a sleeping patient's nasal cavity to assess pharyngeal structures for evidence of obstruction.

This is the only test that can identify a primary epiglottic collapse or a supraglottic collapse.

Table 6.15 AHI and LSAT as parameters of severity of OSA

	AHI	LSAT
Normal	<5	>90
Mild	5–15	>80
Moderate	15–30	70–80
Severe	>30	<70

6.7.1 Sedating Agents

The ideal sedative agent should provide a level of sedation which simulates the natural sleep without affecting the sleep neurophysiology and upper airways collapsing performance. The ideal sedation depth is essential, consisting of a stable pattern of light sedation, defined as the transition from consciousness to unconsciousness (loss of response to verbal stimulation) [18].

The drugs that are commonly used are propofol, midazolam, and dexmedetomidine. The depth of sedation can be assessed with the use of bispectral (BIS) analysis during DISE [18].

The bispectral index (BIS) translates a patient's electroencephalogram (EEG) signals into scaled numbers from 0 (EEG silence) to 100 (fully awake) to reflect the level of consciousness and sedation depth. Loss of consciousness has been reported to occur at BIS values between 60 and 80 [19].

6.7.2 Procedure

Under BIS monitoring, target controlled infusion of one of the sedating agents is performed. Target control infusion with a syringe pump allows better control over sedation. The dosage of the drug is slightly adjusted until the patient starts snoring and reaches a loss of consciousness. Continuous infusion is then given with the pump to maintain the BIS level between 65 and 75 (light sedation).

DISE is performed after the BIS level has remained steady between 65 and 75 for at least 90 sec. [20] A fiberoptic nasal endoscope is passed from the nasal cavity to assess the upper airway. In general, 2 to 3 repeat cycles of snoring, hypoxia, obstruction with apnea, and breakthrough with repeat snoring are observed during DISE to ensure thorough assessment.

6.7.3 Observation/Recordings

DISE findings are recorded according to four anatomic levels: velopharynx, oropharynx, hypopharynx, and larynx.

The severity of velopharynx obstructions following the VOTE classification (velum/oropharynx/tongue base/epiglottis) is recorded as patent/partial/complete obstruction.

The oropharynx, including the tonsils, tongue, and lateral pharyngeal wall, is also evaluated as having patent/partial/complete obstruction.

When the lumen is less than 70% of the expiratory status, partial obstruction is defined. Complete obstruction was recorded when no lumen is seen.

When partial or complete obstruction is noted, the obstruction pattern is classified into circumferential, decreased anteroposterior diameter, or decreased lateral diameter types.

The position of the tongue base is recorded separately in four grades. Tongue base obstruc-

tion is identified when the tongue base pushes the epiglottis backward and causes lumen obstruction. Hypopharynx obstruction is identified when the lateral pharyngeal walls constrict and cause luminal narrowing at the hypopharyngeal level.

The characteristics of the larynx are evaluated in three aspects: anteroposterior prolapse of the epiglottis, lateral folding of the epiglottis, and arytenoid prolapse. When the patients had epiglottis prolapse, epiglottis anteroposterior prolapse that touches the posterior pharyngeal wall (grade 4), or epiglottis folding, they are defined as having larynx obstruction. Multiple-level obstruction is defined when two or more levels are obstructed (Table 6.16).

The simplified version of the above examination findings is the VOTE classification [21] (Table 6.17).

Table 6.16 Reporting of DISE

Velum		Definition
Obstruction Severity	Patent	The airway lumen at end inspiration is greater than 70% of the expiration airway lumen
	Partial obstruction	The airway lumen at end inspiration is lesser than 70% of the expiration airway lumen
	Complete obstruction	No lumen
Obstruction Type	Circumferential	Vertical and transverse diameter collapse proportional to each other
	Anteroposterior	Vertical diameter outweighs the transverse diameter
	Lateral	Transverse diameter outweighs the anteroposterior diameter
Oropharynx		**Definition**
Obstruction Severity	Patent	The airway lumen at end inspiration is greater than 70% of the expiration airway lumen
	Partial obstruction	The airway lumen at end inspiration is lesser than 70% of the expiration airway lumen
	Complete obstruction	No lumen
Obstruction Type	Circumferential	Vertical and transverse diameter collapse proportional to each other
	Anteroposterior	Vertical diameter outweighs the transverse diameter
	Lateral	Transverse diameter outweighs the anteroposterior diameter
Tongue Base		**Defintion**
The position of tongue base is assessed in relation to the valleculae and epiglottis	Grade 1	Valleculae are completely visible
	Grade 2	Valleculae are partially visible
	Grade 3	Tongue base is just touching epiglottis
	Grade 4	Tongue base collapse pushing the epiglottis backward

(continued)

Table 6.16 (continued)

Velum		Definition
Hypopharyx/Epiglottic Obtruction		**Definition**
Hypopharynx obstruction	Yes/No	The lateral pharyngeal walls are collapsing at the level of the hypopharynx
Epiglottis	Grade 1	Vocal cords can be seen completely
	Grade 2	Vocal cords can be seen partially
	Grade 3	Vocal cords cannot be visualized
	Grade 4	Epiglottis touching the posterior pharyngeal wall
Epiglottic collapse	Yes / No	Long tubular epiglottis
Arytenoid collapse	Yes / No	

Table 6.17 VOTE Classification

STRUCTURE	DEGREE OF OBSTRUCTION	CONFIGURATION		
		Antero-Posterior	Lateral	Concentric
Velum				
Oropharynx				
Tongue Base				
Epiglottis				

6.8 Interventional Dise

Nasopharyngeal tubes (NPT) are soft, flexible tubes which are used in airway management. A NPT is placed through the nasal cavity and nasopharynx into the oropharynx until the tip is just beyond the soft palate until the stent opens the palate by separating the soft palate from the posterior pharyngeal wall of the oropharynx.

Having the nasopharyngeal tube during a DISE is used to separate those patients who will respond to isolated oropharyngeal surgery from those patients who will require a multilevel approach.

When a nasopharyngeal tube is placed, it not only improves the palatal level collapse, but also decreases the downstream pharyngeal collapse by reducing the negative pharyngeal pressure. This means that simply addressing only the palate would help the patient [22].

With an NPT, if there is a collapse downstream beyond the palate due of a tongue base hypertrophy, a multilevel surgery must be considered [22].

This will determine whether preventing palatal obstruction with a nasopharyngeal airway alters other sites of airway collapse during DISE [22].

6.9 Dynamic MRI

Dynamic MR imaging can accurately diagnose the cause and level of upper airway narrowing in patients with OSA. It can characterize and anatomically classify the level of narrowing for planning the reparative surgery [23].

MRI evaluation is helpful in determining the level of obstruction, i.e. whether the collapse of the airway is retropalatal or retroglossal or at multiple levels [23].

The main advantage of MRI as compared to other imaging modalities is its ability to perform multiplanar dynamic imaging in the absence of radiation exposure [23].

Nonetheless, an MRI has not become a standard procedure neither in the diagnostic work-up for patients with SDB nor in the management of the disease in terms of surgical or non-surgical treatment. A number of issues remain unresolved: MRI during sleep (especially spontaneous sleep) is possible but not easy to perform and measurements during wakefulness or induced sleep are, to a certain extent, artificial or may simply not reflect clinical conditions [24].

Furthermore, the results of MRI, even when performed during sleep, can only provide information concerning a short period of time and are limited to the supine position. For routine clinical application, the limited availability and the associated costs are additional limiting factors [24].

Although MRI has improved our understanding of SDB, it has not yet become a part of routine clinical evaluation of patients with this condition.

Table 6.18 Evaluation protocol for OSA

Evaluation Protocol
• History: ESS, Stop-Bang Questionnaire, Berlin questionnaire, and Stanford questionnaire.
• Anthropometric Data: Height, Weight, BMI, Neck Circumference.
• Clinical Examination: Nose, Oropharynx [Friedman Tongue Position], Tonsil SIZE, Friedman Staging.
• Polysomnography: Gold Standard, Describes The Severity of OSA, AHI, RDI, Flow Limitation With Snoring, Flow Limitation Without Snoring, Total Snoring Events, Lowest Oxygen Saturation.
• Fibreoptic Nasopharyngoscopy with Muller's Maneuver and end expiratory tongue position: to Identify Site of Obstruction in an Awake Patient.
• Drug Induced Sleep Endoscopy: To Identify Sites of Obstruction after Making the Patient Sleep with Sedating Agents Under Bispectral Index Monitoring to Give More Accurate Results.
• Dynamic MRI: Non-Invasive Method to Identify Sites of Obstruction.

6.10 Apneagraph

An ApneaGraph is a test which measures the airway pressure and airflow simultaneously at different levels in the pharynx and thus identifies the exact segment of airway obstruction and also provides a baseline respiratory parameter which could help in the diagnosis of SDB [25].

In this test, the cardiorespiratory pattern of a patient is recorded at two different sites in the upper airway using a micro-pressure and temperature transducer catheter [25].

By measuring the pressure and airflow (via temperature) it is possible to identify the segment of obstruction during sleep in patients with upper airway obstructions (apnea, hypopnea, and snoring) [25].

6.10.1 Procedure

A pulse oximetry probe is attached to the finger and a Wide-bore catheter is inserted into the nose and placed in the upper esophagus, similar to a nasogastric tube.

There are four transducers (two pressure and two temperature) with one marker probe positioned at the lower border of the soft palate. The marker probe ensures that all the transducers are aligned correctly. The device can be preprogrammed to start at a set time and record for a maximum of 6 h.

This test can be used as a screening tool to identify the presence or absence of OSA. If OSA is identified during an apneagraphy, there are high chances of there being similar findings on the sleep study as well (Table 6.18).

References

1. Johns MW. A new method for measuring daytime sleepiness: the epworth sleepiness scale. Sleep [Internet]. 1991 Nov 1;14(6):540–5. [cited 2021 Feb 22]. Available from: http://academic.oup.com/sleep/article/14/6/540/2742871.
2. Chung F, Abdullah HR, Liao P. STOP-bang questionnaire a practical approach to screen for obstructive sleep apnea. Chest. 2016 Mar 1;149(3):631–8.
3. Hoddes E, Zarcone V, Smythe H, Phillips R, Dement WC. Quantification of sleepiness: a new approach. Psychophysiology [Internet]. 1973 Jul 1;10(4):431–6. [cited 2021 Feb 23]. Available from: http://doi.wiley.com/10.1111/j.1469-8986.1973.tb00801.x.
4. Maurer JT. Early diagnosis of sleep related breathing disorders. GMS Curr Top Otorhinolaryngol Head Neck Surg [Internet]. 2008;7:Doc03. Available from: http://www.ncbi.nlm.nih.gov/pubmed/22073090, http://www.pubmedcentral.nih.gov/articlerender.fcgi?artid=PMC3199834.

5. Kayabekir M. Diagnosis. In: Updates in sleep neurology and obstructive sleep apnea [Working Title] [Internet]. IntechOpen; 2020. [cited 2020 Sep 29]. Available from: https://www.intechopen.com/online-first/diagnosis.

6. Grunstein R, Wilcox I, Yang TS, Gould Y, Hedner J. Snoring and sleep apnoea in men: association with central obesity and hypertenslon. Int J Obes [Internet]. 1993 Sep 1;17(9):533–40. [cited 2020 Sep 29]. Available from: https://europepmc.org/article/med/8220656/reload=0.

7. Abdominal Obesity Measurement Guidelines for Different Ethnic Groups _ Obesity Prevention Source _ Harvard School of Public Health [Internet]. [cited 2020 Sep 29]. Available from: https://www.hsph.harvard.edu/obesity-prevention-source/waist-circumference-guidelines-for-different-ethnic-groups/.

8. Cistulli PA. Craniofacial abnormalities in obstructive sleep apnoea: Implications for treatment. Respirology [Internet]. 1996 Sep 1;1(3):167–74. [cited 2021 Feb 24]. Available from: http://doi.wiley.com/10.1111/j.1440-1843.1996.tb00028.x.

9. Friedman M, Salapatas AM, Bonzelaar LB. Updated Friedman staging system for obstructive sleep apnea. Adv Otorhinolaryngol Basel, Karger. 2017;80:41–8.

10. Tucker WB. A method to describe the pharyngeal airway. Laryngoscope. 2015;125(5):1233–8.

11. Moore KE, Phillips C. A practical method for describing patterns of tongue- base narrowing (modification of Fujita) in awake adult patients with obstructive sleep apnea. J Oral Maxillofac Surg [Internet]. 2002 Dec 11;60(3):252–60. [cited 2020 Sep 29]. Available from: https://linkinghub.elsevier.com/retrieve/pii/S0278239102841246.

12. Lund S, Freeman J. Clinical polysomnography. In: Freidman M, editor. Sleep apnea and snoring. 1st ed. Philadelphia: Saunders Elsevier; 2009. p. 22–32.

13. Le Bon O, Staner L, Hoffmann G, Dramaix M, San Sebastian I, Murphy JR, et al. The first-night effect may last more than one night. J Psychiatr Res. 2001 May 1;35(3):165–72.

14. Shayeb M El, Topfer LA, Stafinski T, Pawluk L, Menon D. Diagnostic accuracy of level 3 portable sleep tests versus level 1 polysomnography for sleep-disordered breathing: a systematic review and meta-analysis. CMAJ [Internet]. 2014 Jan 7;186(1):E25. [cited 2021 Feb 25]. Available from: https://www.ncbi.nlm.nih.gov/pmc/articles/PMC3883848/.

15. Sabil A, Eberhard A, Baconnier P, Benchetrit G. A physical model of inspiratory flow limitation in awake healthy subjects. In: Advances in experimental medicine and biology. New York: Kluwer Academic/Plenum Publishers; 2004. p. 211–6.

16. Deenadayal DS, Vidyasagar D, Bommakanti V. Can number of sites of obstruction be predicted on a level 3 home sleep study? Int J Otolaryngol Head Neck Surg. 2018;07(03):80–7.

17. Croft CB, Pringle M. Sleep nasendoscopy: a technique of assessment in snoring and obstructive sleep apnoea. Clin Otolaryngol [Internet]. 1991 Oct;16(5):504–9. [cited 2021 Feb 25]. Available from: https://pubmed.ncbi.nlm.nih.gov/1742903/.

18. Kotecha B, De Vito A. Drug induced sleep endoscopy: Its role in evaluation of the upper airway obstruction and patient selection for surgical and nonsurgical treatment [Internet]. J Thorac Dis. 2018;10:S40–7. [cited 2021 Feb 25]. AME Publishing Company. Available from: https://www.ncbi.nlm.nih.gov/pmc/articles/PMC5803054/.

19. Lo YL, Ni YL, Wang TY, Lin TY, Li HY, White DP, et al. Bispectral index in evaluating effects of sedation depth on drug-induced sleep endoscopy. J Clin Sleep Med [Internet]. 2015;11(9):1011–20. [cited 2021 Feb 25]. Available from: https://www.ncbi.nlm.nih.gov/pmc/articles/PMC4543245/.

20. Yl L, Yl N, Wang TY, Ty L, Li HY, Dp W, et al. Bispectral index in evaluating effects of sedation depth on drug-induced sleep endoscopy. J Clin Sleep Med [Internet]. 2015;11(9):1011–1020. [cited 2020 Sep 29]. Available from: https://doi.org/10.5664/jcsm.5016.

21. Kezirian EJ, Hohenhorst W, De Vries N. Drug-induced sleep endoscopy: the vote classification. Eur Arch Oto-Rhino-Laryngology [Internet]. 2011 Aug 26;268(8):1233–6. [cited 2020 Sep 29]. Available from: https://link.springer.com/article/10.1007/s00405-011-1633-8.

22. Victores AJ, Olson K, Takashima M. Interventional Drug-Induced Sleep Endoscopy: A novel technique to guide surgical planning for obstructive sleep apnea. J Clin Sleep Med [Internet]. 2017 [cited 2021 Feb 25];13(2):169–74. Available from: https://www.ncbi.nlm.nih.gov/pmc/articles/PMC5263071/.

23. Bhawna, Santosham R, Anand S, Joseph S. Role of dynamic MR imaging in obstructive sleep apnoea. Indian J Otolaryngol Head Neck Surg [Internet]. 2008 Mar;60(1):25–9. [cited 2021 Feb 25]. Available from: https://www.ncbi.nlm.nih.gov/pmc/articles/PMC3450703/.

24. Stuck BA, Maurer JT. Airway evaluation in obstructive sleep apnea. In: Friedman M, editor. Sleep apnea and snoring. Philadelphia: Saunders Elsevier; 2009. p. 11–21.

25. Singh A, Al-Reefy H, Hewitt R, Kotecha B. Evaluation of ApneaGraph in the diagnosis of sleep-related breathing disorders. Eur Arch Otorhinolaryngol. 2008;265:1489–94.

There are numerous options for the management of a patient with OSA. These treatments range from non-invasive modifications to PAP therapy and surgeries. The selection of a treatment option for a patient is complex given the range of variability that could occur in a patient's anatomy and physiology and also the severity of the disease. In addition to these factors, certain other factors also influence the treatment options like the patient's preference and compliance and the associated co-morbidities. In this chapter, the non-surgical management of OSA will be discussed.

7.1 Medical Treatments

Medical therapy with decongestants, intranasal steroids, anti-histamines, and antileukotrienes has demonstrated a favorable sleep pattern and thus lead to an improvement in the quality of life.

Modafinil: Modafinil is a wake-promoting drug licensed to treat residual sleepiness in CPAP-treated OSA. We hypothesized that modafinil may effectively treat sleepiness in untreated mild to moderate OSA [1].

Medical therapy can be used in conjunction with PAP therapy or other forms of conservative therapies like mandibular advancement devices for the management of OSA.

7.2 Obesity Management

Obesity management is one of the key aspects in the treatment of OSA. There is reasonably well-established evidence that treatment of obesity improves OSA. Weight loss has shown to improve the oxygenation and reduce respiratory events in patients with OSA [2].

Lifestyle modification essentially consists of three important components

1. Dietary therapy.

    Intermittent fasting is an eating plan that switches between fasting and eating on a regular schedule. With intermittent fasting you only eat during a specific time. Fasting for a certain number of hours each day or eating just one meal a couple days a week can help your body burn fat.
2. Physical activity.
3. Behavioral therapy.

Adjuvant pharmacotherapy maybe used in patients in whom lifestyle modifications have been unsuccessful or in patients with BMI > 30 kg/m^2 [3]. Even if pharmacotherapy is initiated, the patients must be motivated to sustain a dietary modification and regular physical exercise in order to see balanced and sustainable weight loss results. There are various drug thera-

© The Author(s), under exclusive license to Springer Nature Singapore Pte Ltd. 2022
D. S. Deenadayal, V. Bommakanti, *Management of Snoring and Obstructive Sleep Apnea*,
https://doi.org/10.1007/978-981-16-6620-9_7

pies that can be used. Depending on the mechanism of action, they are classified into centrally acting drugs which reduce the satiety, peripherally acting drugs like Orlistat which increase the metabolism and the endocannabinoid system which causes endocrinological changes to decrease the appetite [3].

Weight loss surgery—Bariatric surgery may be considered in patients with severe obesity BMI > 40 kg/m2.

7.3 Use of Oral Appliances

The concept of using oral appliances to relieve upper airway obstruction was first reported in the 1930s and applied to OSA more than 30 years ago [4]. In the recent years, there has been an increasing interest in oral appliances because of the high prevalence of OSA and recognition of the limitations of PAP therapy and surgical therapy [4].

A multidisciplinary approach is required to effectively manage a patient who has OSA with an oral appliance. It is necessary to have a dental evaluation which includes assessment of suitability for oral appliance therapy, device selection, and fitting.

7.4 Oral Appliance Therapy

Oral appliances are an effective therapy for OSA and work by enlarging and stabilizing the pharyngeal airway to prevent breathing obstructions during sleep [5].

PAP therapy is highly efficacious in preventing pharyngeal collapse but there is a subset of patients who are non-compliant thus creating the need for alternate treatment options.

Oral appliances can be broadly classified as devices that protrude the tongue (tongue retaining devices, TRD) and devices that advance the lower jaw (commonly termed mandibular advancement splints or devices) [5].

There are more than 150 devices with FDA approval for the treatment of snoring and OSA patients, but there is a debate about the efficacy of these different devices [5].

As per clinical guidelines, customized devices which are titratable should be dispensed by a qualified dentist. Non-customized devices offer poor results as compared to customized devices [6].

In recent years, devices are emerging which rely on computer-aided design or computer-aided manufacturing technology. Instead of the traditional impressions, digital intraoral scans can now be used to design appliances, and digital manufacturing techniques are increasingly being used. These can streamline the process and result in more rapid access to treatment and better fit of appliances, which could improve acceptance and efficacy [5].

7.5 Tongue Retaining Device

The tongue retaining device functions by holding the tongue in a forward position by means of a suction bulb. This prevents the tongue from collapsing during sleep and obstructing the airway [7].

7.6 Mandibular Advancement Devices [Mad]

MADs are the most commonly used oral appliances and recommended in the treatment of snoring and mild to moderate OSAHS patients [8], but they were rarely used in patients with severe OSAHS, especially in those with persistent OSAHS condition even after surgical treatment.

There are multiple MAD designs but preferred are the devices which intend to protrude the mandible, increase the tension of soft tissues of the soft palate, lateral pharyngeal walls, and the tongue, and thus improve the airway patency.

A MAD device can be considered as a treatment option for patients with a persistent VP obstruction even after surgery, if they are unable to tolerate CPAP, refuse PAP therapy or a more invasive surgery. Thus, MAD might be an effective and feasible treatment for non-responding patients after upper airway surgery [9].

7.6.1 Myofunctional Therapy/Oral Facial Myofunctional Therapy

Orofacial myofunctional therapy (OMT) is a modality of treatment for children and adults with obstructive sleep apnea (OSA) which promotes changes in the musculature of the upper airways [10].

7.6.2 Principle

The principle behind myofunctional therapy is that working the orofacial muscles with targeted exercises can help to tone and strengthen the tissue and train it to remain in place thus keeping the airway unobstructed.

OMT is based on exercises that favor sensitivity, proprioception, mobility, coordination, and strength of orofacial structures, as well as promote an appropriate performance of respiration, mastication, deglutition, and speech [10].

7.6.3 Indications

Children may benefit from myofunction if they.

- have been diagnosed with mild/moderate OSA,
- have been snoring or mouth breathing,
- have large tonsils with lax tongue obstructing the airway.

In adults, myofunctional therapy is used less often as it is less effective. It can be used as an adjunct to other procedure or may be used post palatal or tongue base surgery if they have mild symptoms of snoring.

7.6.4 Technique

The most comprehensive MT exercises are described by Guimaraes et al. and they involve the soft palate, tongue, and facial muscles thus addressing stomatognathic functions [11]. For soft palate exercises, patients pronounce oral vowel sounds either continuously (isometric exercises) or intermittently (isotonic exercises) [11, 12]. Tongue exercises include moving the tongue along the superior and lateral surfaces of the teeth, positioning the tongue tip against the anterior aspect of the hard palate, pressing the entire tongue against the hard and soft palate, and forcing the tongue onto the floor of the mouth [11, 12]. Facial exercises address the lip (i.e., contraction and relaxation of the orbicularis oris), buccinators (i.e., suction movements and application of intraoral finger pressure against the buccinator muscles), and jaw muscles (i.e., lateral jaw movements) [11, 12]. In addition, stomatognathic functions are addressed by instructing patients to inhale nasally and exhale orally without and then with balloon inflation, and performing specific swallowing and chewing exercises (i.e., swallowing with the teeth clenched together, tongue positioned in the palate and without contraction of perioral muscles; alternating chewing sides) [11, 12]. Now we have various devices that condition and strengthen oral and tongue muscles [11, 13].

Myofunctional therapy can be incorporated as a primary modality of therapy in children who may be susceptible to OSA in their adulthood. It can be used as an adjunct to various other therapies in the treatment of adult sleep apnea [11].

References

1. Chapman JL, Kempler L, Chang CL, Williams SC, Sivam S, Wong KKH, et al. Modafinil improves daytime sleepiness in patients with mild to moderate obstructive sleep apnoea not using standard treatments: a randomised placebo-controlled crossover trial. Thorax [Internet] 2014 Mar;69(3):274–279. [cited 2020 Oct 4]. Available from: https://pubmed.ncbi.nlm.nih.gov/24287166/.
2. Strobel RJ, Rosen RC. Obesity and weight loss in obstructive sleep apnea: a critical review. Sleep. 1996;19(2):104–15.
3. Kushner RF. Obesity management. In: Friedman M, editor. Sleep apnea and snoring. Philadelphia: Saunders Elsevier; 2009. p. 51–9.
4. Vanderveken OM, Braem MJ, De Backer WA, Van De Heyning PH. The concept of using oral appliances to relieve upper airway obstruction was first reported in the 1930s and applied to OSA more than 30 years ago.

[Internet]. Minerva Pneumologica. 2011;50:237–45. [cited 2020 Sep 29]. Available from: https://www. uptodate.com/contents/oral-appliances-in-the-treatment-of-obstructive-sleep-apnea-in-adults.

5. Sutherland K, Cistulli PA. Oral appliance therapy for obstructive sleep Apnoea: state of the art. J Clin Med [Internet]. 2019 Dec 2;8(12):2121. [cited 2021 Feb 26]. Available from: https://www.ncbi.nlm.nih.gov/ pmc/articles/PMC6947472/.

6. Vanderveken OM, Devolder A, Marklund M, Boudewyns AN, Braem MJ, Okkerse W, et al. Comparison of a custom-made and a thermoplastic oral appliance for the treatment of mild sleep apnea. Am J Respir Crit Care Med [Internet]. 2008 Jul 15;178(2):197–202. [cited 2021 Feb 26]. Available from: https://pubmed.ncbi.nlm.nih.gov/17673699/.

7. Miyazaki S, Kikuchi M. Oral appliance and craniofacial problems. In: Friedman M, editor. Snoring and sleep apnea. Philadelphia: Saunders Elsevier; 2009. p. 72–9.

8. Basyuni S, Barabas M, Quinnell T. An update on mandibular advancement devices for the treatment of obstructive sleep apnoea hypopnoea syndrome [Internet]. J Thorac Dis. 2018;10:S48–56. AME Publishing Company. [cited 2020 Oct 3]. Available from: https://www.ncbi.nlm.nih.gov/pmc/articles/PMC5803051/?report=abstract.

9. Luo H, Tang X, Xiong Y, Meng L, Yi H, Yin S. Efficacy and mechanism of mandibular advance-ment devices for persistent sleep apnea after surgery: a prospective study. J Otolaryngol – Head Neck Surg [Internet]. 2016 Nov 3 [cited 2020 Oct 3];45(1):1–8. Available from: https://www.ncbi.nlm.nih.gov/pmc/articles/PMC5096336/?report=abstract.

10. de Felício CM, Dias FV da S, Trawitzki LVV. Obstructive sleep apnea: Focus on myofunctional therapy [Internet]. Nat Sci Sleep. 2018;10:271–86. Dove Medical Press Ltd. [cited 2020 Oct 3]. Available from: https://www.ncbi.nlm.nih.gov/pmc/articles/PMC6132228/?report=abstract.

11. Camacho M, Certal V, Abdullatif J, Zaghi S, Ruoff CM, Capasso R, et al. Myofunctional therapy to treat obstructive sleep apnea: A systematic review and meta-analysis. Sleep [Internet]. 2015 May 1;38(5):669–75. [cited 2020 Oct 3]. Available from: https://academic. oup.com/sleep/article/38/5/669/2416863.

12. Guimarães KC, Drager LF, Genta PR, Marcondes BF, Lorenzi-Filhoy G. Effects of oropharyngeal exercises on patients with moderate obstructive sleep apnea syndrome. Am J Respir Crit Care Med [Internet]. 2009;179(10):962–6. [cited 2020 Oct 3]. Available from: www.clinicaltrials.gov.

13. Suzuki H, Watanabe A, Akihiro Y, Takao M, Ikematsu T, Kimoto S, et al. Pilot study to assess the potential of oral myofunctional therapy for improving respiration during sleep. J Prosthodont Res. 2013 Jul 1;57(3):195–9.

OSA is a disorder that needs to be evaluated and managed by a team of specialists and the role of dentistry in sleep disorders is becoming more significant, especially in co-managing patients with simple snoring and mild to moderate OSA.

The dental professional has the opportunity to assist patients at a variety of levels, starting with the recognition of a sleep-related disorder by identifying the changes that occur in the oral cavity, referring patients to a physician for further evaluation, and assisting in the management of sleep disorders by various surgical and non-surgical methods of treatment.

The dental perspectives of OSA are described in this chapter.

- Pre-treatment dental assessment is essential in the management of patients with OSA.

  This includes.

- Dental history.

In children, it is essential to screen habits which play an important role in the development of stomatognathic system.

The habits may be classified as.

- Habits which prevent OSA like nasal breathing
- Habits which increase the risk of OSA, like thumb sucking, use of pacifiers, bottle feeding, mouth breathing, nail biting, pencil biting, tongue thrusting, and bruxism [1].

8.1 Association of Dentition/Chewing Habits and OSA

Presence of dentition maintains a good lower face height and a gonial angle [Angle that jaw line makes].

The gonial angle is increased in partially edentulous, compared to dentate individuals, but not as greatly as for those individuals who are fully edentulous. A large gonial angle is found to be associated with obstructive sleep apnea [2, 3].

There are changes in the masticatory muscles that accompany partial as well as complete loss of the teeth. The loss of tone and decreased strength of the masticatory muscles also result partially in decreasing the stability of mandible and the oral airway.

Maintenance of occlusal support protects against atrophy of masseter muscle fiber thickness and volume, especially in the premolar region [4].

Dentures restore the vertical dimension of occlusion, lower facial height, retropharyngeal and posterior airway spaces, and peak inspiratory flow rates [5].

Chewing is an important habit that also to a certain extent attribute to OSA. Decreased chewing due to improper dentition or malocclusion leads to a bolus which is more semi-solid in consistency. This bolus is not digested well and results in weight gain on a long term thus contributing to obesity and OSA.

8.2   Oral Examination

Often in patients with OSA, the changes that occur in the tooth and the periodontal region are often missed and have received less attention.

It is important to assess the oral status as part of routine evaluation in patients with OSA [6].

In patients with snoring/OSA there is associated.

- Posterior teeth grinded/worn out—Signs of bruxism,
- Flat cusps with loss of key of occlusion which makes lower jaw slide back (Fig. 8.1).

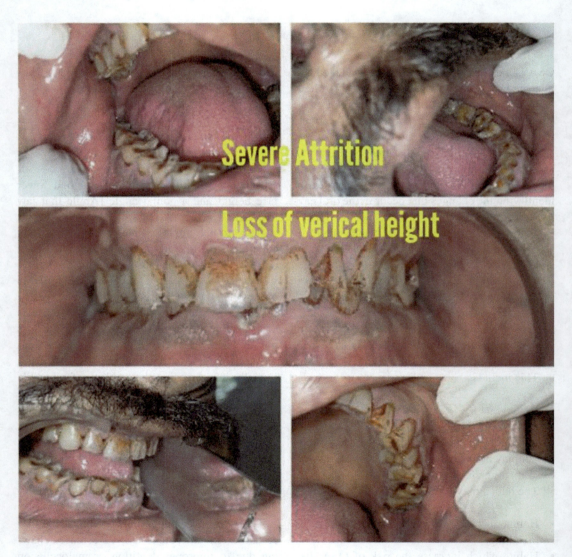

Fig. 8.1 Clinical picture of severe attrition and loss of vertical height

Other examination findings to consider are.

- Incompetent lips/malocclusion/periodontitis.
- Narrow dental arch—V shaped maxillary arch.
- High arched palate.
- Increased anterior face height—long face.
- The tongue placed low on mandibular teeth.
- Steep mandibular plane angle.
- Retrognathic mandible.
- The dental, skeletal midlines, and temporomandibular joint (TMJ) status have to be recorded prior to treatment planning.

8.3   Treatment Options

The treatment options for patients with OSA is based on the severity of OSA, preference of the patient, patient's general health, and the experience of the team.

From a dentist's perspective treatment options include.

8.4   Oral Appliances

Oral devices are basically thermoplastic materials with retainers and supports and are usually tailored as per the needs of the patient. They can be classified as follows:

8.5   For Children

Myofunctional Appliance: These devices are used to guide the eruption of teeth and development of jaw, to allow proper positioning of them in the oral cavity. These devices can be given in children as young as 3 years.

They are given in two phases.

- PHASE-I.

  In the first phase a soft (silicon material) appliance is given with a labial bow to guide proper eruption and development of dentition. This device also prevents the inward movement of the palatal and tongue muscles during

the childhood thus allowing development of a functional airway.
- PHASE-II.

  Appliance is similar except that it is a little harder (polyurethane material) so as to assist development of upper and lower jaws correctly and achieve a correct bite.

Instructions for use:

- Child is advised to wear it for one hour when conscious/active and then slowly over the entire night.
- To keep the lips closed and practice NOSE BREATHING.
- Tongue to be placed on its tongue rest.

8.6   For Adults

These devices are recommended in patients with primary snoring or mild to moderate sleep apnea. They can also be used in conjunction with other modalities of treatment like PAP therapy or in patients with residual OSA post-surgery.

(a) Mandibular repositioning or advancement devices (MRD/MAD) which may be titratable, e.g. Herbst appliance/snoreguard/silencer.

They function by engaging one or both of the dental arches to modify mandibular protrusion [7].

They have to be snapped into the upper and lower jaw thus advancing the mandible anteriorly (Fig. 8.2).

(b) Tongue repositioning or retaining devices (TRD), e.g., SnorEx.

A tongue retaining device is a custom-made soft acrylic appliance that covers the upper and lower teeth and has an anterior plastic bulb. It uses negative suction pressure to hold the tongue in a forward position thus increasing the retroglossal space and also stabilize the mandible and hyoid bone [7].

These devices, reverse pharyngeal obstruction both at the level of the oropharynx and the hypopharynx, thereby enlarging

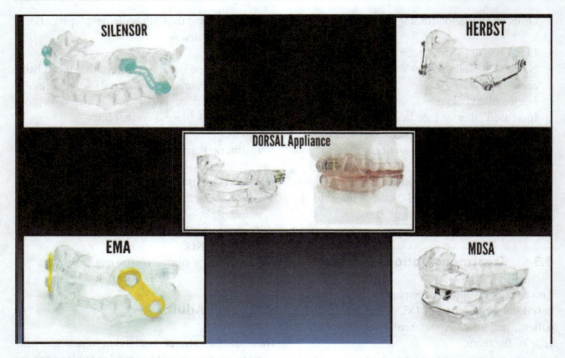

Fig. 8.2 Mandibular Repositioning Devices

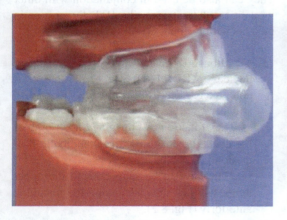

Fig. 8.3 Tongue Retaining Device

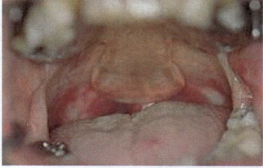

Fig. 8.4 Soft palate lift

the airway and reducing snoring and the related apnea [7] (Fig. 8.3).

(c) Soft-palate lifters.

These devices lift the soft palate, and are useful in patients with weak palatopharyngeus muscle [8, 9] (Fig. 8.4).

(d) A combination of oral appliance and CPAP in the new products delivers pressurized air directly into the oral cavity and eliminates the use of head gear or nasal mask and avoids the problems of air leaks and the claustrophobia associated with CPAP treatment [7] (Fig. 8.5).

Factors which predict the response to oral appliances [10].

– Age of the patient—young adults are often reluctant to the use of appliances.

– Change in weight over 12 months or weight loss,

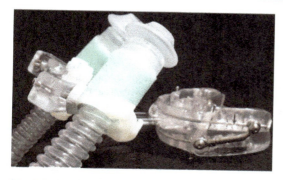

Fig. 8.5 Oral appliance with CPAP

- Lowering of BMI < 25 percent obesity—weight loss results in improper fitting of the appliance and thus result in non-compliance,
- Initial severity of the AHI scores [11–21],
- Supine sleeping position,
- Patient's tolerance and motivation.

8.7 Advantages

- Non-invasive.
- Not very expansive.
- Easy to use and handle and can be carried anywhere along with patient.

8.8 Disadvantages/Complications

- Dental malocclusion.
- TMJ pain and TMJ dislocation.
- Excessive salivation, tongue dryness, tooth pain, posterior open bite, and insomnia.

References

1. Grippaudo C, Paolantonio EG, Antonini G, Saulle R, La Torre G, Deli R. Associazione fra abitudini viziate, respirazione orale e malocclusione. Acta Otorhinolaryngol Ital. 2016;36(5):386–94.
2. Anderson S, Alsufyani N, Isaac A, Gazzaz M, El-Hakim H. Correlation between gonial angle and dynamic tongue collapse in children with snoring/sleep disordered breathing – an exploratory pilot study. J Otolaryngol – Head Neck Surg [Internet]. 2018 Jun 4;47(1). [cited 2020 Oct 3]. Available from: https://www.ncbi.nlm.nih.gov/pmc/articles/PMC5987664/?report=abstract.
3. Lowe AA, Santamaria JD, Fleetham JA, Price C. Facial morphology and obstructive sleep apnea. Am J Orthod Dentofac Orthop [Internet]. 1986 Dec;90(6):484–91. [cited 2020 Oct 3]. Available from: https://linkinghub.elsevier.com/retrieve/pii/0889540686901083.
4. Sanders AE, Akinkugbe AA, Slade GD, Essick GK. Tooth loss and obstructive sleep apnea signs and symptoms in the US population. Sleep Breath [Internet]. 2016 Sep 1;20(3):1095–102. [cited 2020 Oct 3]. Available from: https://www.ncbi.nlm.nih.gov/pmc/articles/PMC4947024/?report=abstract.
5. Gupta P, Thombare R, Pakhan AJ, Singhal S. Cephalometric evaluation of the effect of complete dentures on retropharyngeal space and its effect on Spirometric values in altered vertical dimension. ISRN Dent [Internet]. 2011;2011:1–9. [cited 2020 Oct 3]. Available from: https://www.ncbi.nlm.nih.gov/pmc/articles/PMC3168939/?report=abstract.
6. Miyazaki S, Kikuchi M. Oral appliance and craniofacial problems. In: Friedman M, editor. Snoring and sleep apnea. Philadelphia: Saunders Elsevier; 2009. p. 72–9.
7. Raghavan R, ShajahanP A, MonishaV S. Management of obstructive sleep apnoea: a review article. Int J Med Sci Clin Invent. 2018;5:3844–7.
8. Bhalla G, Arya D, Chand P, Singh K, Tripathi S. Management of obstructive sleep apnea with a palatal lift prosthesis. Int J Stomatol Occlusion Med [Internet]. 2013 Sep 17;6(3):101–5. [cited 2021 Feb 27]. Available from: https://link.springer.com/article/10.1007/s12548-013-0088-5
9. Raj N, Raj V, Aeran H. Interim palatal lift prosthesis as a constituent of multidisciplinary approach in the treatment of velopharyngeal incompetence. J Adv Prosthodont [Internet]. 2012;4(4):243–7. [cited 2021 Feb 27]. Available from: https://www.ncbi.nlm.nih.gov/pmc/articles/PMC3517964/.
10. Chan AS, Cistulli PA. Oral appliance treatment of obstructive sleep apnea: an update. Curr Opin Pulm Med [Internet]. 2009 Nov;15(6):591–6. [cited 2021 Feb 27]. Available from: https://journals.lww.com/00063198-200911000-00011.
11. Konecny T, Kara T, Somers VK. Obstructive sleep apnea and hypertension: an update. Hypertension [Internet]. 2014 Feb;63(2):203. [cited 2020 Sep 6]. Available from: https://www.ncbi.nlm.nih.gov/pmc/articles/PMC4249687/.
12. Kohli P, Balachandran JS, Malhotra A. Obstructive sleep apnea and the risk for cardiovascular disease [Internet]. Curr Atheroscler Rep. 2011;13:138–46. NIH Public Access. [cited 2020 Sep 6]. Available from: https://www.ncbi.nlm.nih.gov/pmc/articles/PMC4332589/?report=abstract.
13. Jean-Louis G, Brown CD, Zizi F, Ogedegbe G, Boutin-Foster C, Gorga J, et al. Cardiovascular disease risk reduction with sleep apnea treatment [Internet]. Expert Rev Cardiovasc Ther. 2010;8:995–1005. Expert Reviews Ltd. [cited 2021 Feb 19].

Available from: https://www.ncbi.nlm.nih.gov/pmc/articles/PMC4234108/.

14. Gonzaga C, Bertolami A, Bertolami M, Amodeo C, Calhoun D. Obstructive sleep apnea, hypertension and cardiovascular diseases. J Hum Hypertens [Internet]. 2015;29(12):705–12. Available from: http://www.ncbi.nlm.nih.gov/pubmed/25761667

15. Lattimore JDL, Celermajer DS, Wilcox I. Obstructive sleep apnea and cardiovascular disease. J Am Coll Cardiol [Internet]. 2003 May 7;41(9):1429–37. [cited 2020 Sep 8]. Available from: https://www.onlinejacc.org/content/41/9/1429.

16. McNicholas WT, Bonsignore MR. Sleep apnoea as an independent risk for cardiovascular disease: current evidence, basic mechanisms and research priorities. Eur Respir J [Internet]. 2007 Jan 1;29(1):156–78. [cited 2020 Sep 8]. Available from: https://erj.ersjournals.com/content/29/1/156.

17. Kohli P, Balachandran JS, Malhotra A. Obstructive sleep apnea and the risk for cardiovascular disease. Curr Atheroscler Rep. 2011;13:138–46.

18. Cross NE, Memarian N, Duffy SL, Paquola C, LaMonica H, D'Rozario A, et al. Structural brain correlates of obstructive sleep apnoea in older adults at risk for dementia. Eur Respir J [Internet]. 2018 Jul 1;52(1):1800740. [cited 2020 Sep 8]. Available from: https://doi.org/10.1183/13993003.00740-2018.

19. Goldstein AN, Walker MP. The role of sleep in emotional brain function [Internet]. Annu Rev Clin Psychol. 2014;10:679–708. Annual Reviews Inc. [cited 2020 Sep 8]. Available from: https://www.ncbi.nlm.nih.gov/pmc/articles/PMC4286245/?report=abstract.

20. Gupta MA, Simpson FC. Obstructive sleep apnea and psychiatric disorders: a systematic review. J Clin Sleep Med. 2015;11:165–75. American Academy of Sleep Medicine

21. Framnes SN, Arble DM. The bidirectional relationship between obstructive sleep apnea and metabolic disease [Internet]. Front Endocrinol. 2018;9:440. Frontiers Media S.A. [cited 2020 Sep 8]. Available from: https://www.ncbi.nlm.nih.gov/pmc/articles/PMC6087747/?report=abstract.

Positive airway pressure (PAP) is the primary modality of treatment in various sleep-disordered breathing disorders like obstructive sleep apnea, central sleep apnea, and sleep-related hypoventilation. All patients must be allowed to try this therapy as a treatment option and surgical intervention must be considered only in case of failure of PAP therapy.

There are various devices for delivering positive airway pressure, the most common being continuous positive airway pressure (CPAP) which maintains a continuous level of positive airway pressure in a spontaneously breathing patient. Other forms that provide non-invasive positive pressure ventilation include bilevel positive airway pressure (BiPAP), adaptive servo ventilation (SV), and volume-assured pressure support (VAPS).

PAP equipment involves three basic parts: a device with a motor, a mask that covers either the mouth or the nose, or both and a tube that connects the device to the mask.

9.1 Type of Devices

9.1.1 CPAP

CPAP maintains a continuous PAP throughout inspiration and expiration. Auto adjusting (Auto) CPAP can gradually increase or decrease the pressure based on the respiratory events, but it maintains the same pressure throughout the respiratory cycle.

Indication: This device is useful in patients who need assisted pressure support only during rapid eye movement (REM) sleep or in supine position but cannot tolerate the high pressure through the entire night.

Most CPAP devices allow for pressure settings between 4 and 20 cm·H_2O [1]. The goal of CPAP is to increase the upper airway pressure enough to open the airway, which may collapse during inspiration. Typically, the pressure is set to prevent hypopnea, apnea, snoring, flow limitation, and arousals.

The aim of Auto CPAP is to adjust the pressure in response to respiratory events.

If a patient enters REM sleep or changes position, the degree of obstruction may suddenly increase and by the time the device is able to adjust to the needed pressure, the patient may have had desaturations or arousals [1]. Auto CPAP is most often able to recognize these variations and make adjustments as per the respiratory efforts of the patient.

Titration of a PAP can be done in the lab or at home. In the lab, it can be done through a split night titration where PAP therapy is administered half way through a polysomnography. For those who want a home titration, an auto titrating PAP machine is provided to the patient for use for a

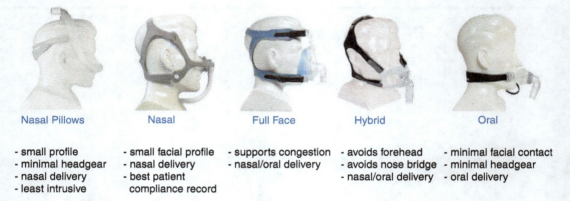

Nasal Pillows	Nasal	Full Face	Hybrid	Oral
- small profile	- small facial profile	- supports congestion	- avoids forehead	- minimal facial contact
- minimal headgear	- nasal delivery	- nasal/oral delivery	- avoids nose bridge	- minimal headgear
- nasal delivery	- best patient		- nasal/oral delivery	- oral delivery
- least intrusive	compliance record			

Fig. 9.1 Various masks used for CPAP or BiPAP devices

period of 3 to 7 days. The machine is then returned to the physician for assessment of the reports.

9.1.2 BiPAP

BiPAP provides a higher pressure during inspiration and lower pressure during expiration. This may improve tolerance and help with ventilation. A backup rate can be added to give a breath with weak or absent respiratory effort.

AutoBiPAP may adjust either the expiratory positive airway pressure (EPAP) and inspiratory positive airway pressure (IPAP) with a fixed pressure support (PS) or may adjust them independently.

BiPAP provides a higher pressure during inhalation and lower pressure during exhalation. Pressures generally range from an EPAP minimum of four to an IPAP maximum of 25–30. Most devices use a flow trigger to determine when to change to IPAP. The trigger is set above zero flow to sense a significant patient effort [1].

9.1.3 Masks

It is believed that the efficacy of PAP therapy depends on the mask [2]. There are various types of masks available and no single mask can be said to be suitable for all patients. Masks are classified into three types—nasal masks, oral masks, and oronasal masks. The patients must be allowed to try out an assortment of masks during the PAP trial, thus allowing them to choose what suits them best.

For improving compliance and to assure lesser discomfort, silicon based masks are available which are soft and less traumatic (Fig. 9.1).

9.2   Servo Ventilation

It is a bilevel system that continuously changes the inspiratory PS on a breath- by-breath basis in order to achieve a target ventilation or flow for a more constant breathing pattern, especially in the treatment of periodic breathing or Cheyne–Stokes respiration (CSR) [1].

9.3   Volume Assisted Pressure Support

Volume-assured pressure support (VAPS) is a variable bilevel PAP that allows the target volume or ventilation to be programmed, which allows more control of ventilation in patients with chronic obstructive pulmonary disease (COPD), neuromuscular disorders, or obesity, who may need different pressure support levels at different times [1].

9.4 Compliance with PAP

Most patients take a trial once or twice with the mask and the machine only to pronounce that they are uncomfortable with the therapy. This does not constitute a CPAP failure. The physician and technician must encourage patients to learn how to use the machine and also try different masks if they feel uncomfortable with a certain type.

The first night with PAP is often the most difficult and the technician must follow up with the patient in order to identify the problems and help the patient with them.

Current trends define compliance as 4 hours a night as an average over *all* nights observed [1, 3].

CPAP compliance issues can be divided into the following:

- *Acceptance:* enduring the use of the CPAP machine in order that the optimum pressure can be adjusted;
- *Prescription*: actually starting with the therapy;
- *Adherence*: continuation of the treatment; and.
- *Tolerance*: permanent acceptance of treatment without adverse reactions. Failure includes refusal of the device, withdrawal directly after initiating treatment, or failure to reduce the apnea/hypopnea index (AHI) sufficiently.

Reasons for CPAP failure as shown in various studies are decreased nasal passage, dry eyes, claustrophobia, leakage of the mask, no effect, cannot fall asleep with it and removal during sleep without awakening.

To improve compliance, there are various methods but the two most commonly used approaches are

1. The patient should be familiarized with how the mask feels. They can be initially asked to use the mask in the evening and eventually sleep with it on. PAP can be added at a later stage only when the patient is completely comfortable with the mask.
2. PAP compliance can be increased by initially starting with low pressure and then gradually increasing it to the therapeutic level in a couple of days.

For patients who complain of a dry feeling in the nose, a humidifier may be used.

A surgeon must try to identify any possible cause for upper airway obstruction that is reducing the compliance of PAP and correct it so as to improve compliance. If there is any factor causing an obstructing in the airway, the surgeon must correct it so as to improve the compliance with PAP.

If there is a nasal mask PAP therapy non-compliance, then a cause in the nose like DNS/hypertrophic turbinate/polyps or adenoids must be looked into, while if there is an oronasal mask PAP non-compliance, then epiglottic collapse, supraglottic collapse, or a bilateral abductor palsy must be checked for.

References

1. Johnson KG, Johnson DC. Treatment of sleep-disordered breathing with positive airway pressure devices: Technology update [Internet]. Med Devices: Evidence Res. 2015;8:425–37. Dove Medical Press Ltd. [cited 2020 Oct 3]. Available from: https://www.ncbi.nlm.nih.gov/pmc/articles/PMC4629962/?report=abstract.
2. Genta PR, Kaminska M, Edwards BA, Ebben MR, Krieger AC, Tamisier R, et al. The importance of mask selection on continuous positive airway pressure outcomes for obstructive sleep apnea an Official American Thoracic Society Workshop Report [Internet]. Annals of the Am Thorac Soc. 2020;17:1177–85. Available from: https://www.atsjournals.org/doi/10.1513/AnnalsATS.202007-864ST.
3. Ravesloot MJL, De Vries N. Reliable calculation of the efficacy of non- surgical and surgical treatment of obstructive sleep apnea revisited. Sleep [Internet]. 2011 Jan 1;34(1):105–10. [cited 2021 Feb 27]. Available from: https://www.ncbi.nlm.nih.gov/pmc/articles/PMC3001787/.

10.1 Patient Selection for Surgery

In patients with sleep-disordered breathing, it is necessary to be sure who needs surgery, when do they need surgery, and what type of a surgery is the most appropriate for the patient's clinical condition.

After a thorough evaluation and identifying the levels of obstruction, surgical procedures are tailored to the requirements of the patient. The treatment protocol varies from person to person.

It is important to first determine the patients concerns and complaints and also identify if there are underlying medical comorbidities contributing to the current status of the patient.

In adult OSA, non-surgical management like using a PAP therapy, obesity management, and oral devices must be considered prior to surgery. Patients who fail to comply with these measures must be then considered for surgery.

Proper screening and evaluation are vital prior to the surgery to achieve good outcomes and to reduce the possibility of postoperative complications.

As mentioned in prior chapter, a polysomnography is critical in the evaluation of a patient. No patient must undergo a surgery without a prior PSG.

In addition to other investigation that identify anatomical levels of obstruction like fiberoptic laryngopharyngoscopy or drug induced sleep endoscopy, a comprehensive panel of tests must be recommended. These tests include CBP, metabolic parameter, ECG, chest X-ray, and other investigations that are done as routine to assess the fitness of the patient for surgery.

10.2 Rationale and Indications for Surgery in OSA

10.2.1 Aim

The aim of surgery is to achieve an outcome that makes patient symptom free and be able to achieve outcomes that are comparable to a CPAP.

Additionally, the goal is to improve quality of life, reduce the risk or cardiac and cerebrovascular or other medical events and increase the longevity.

10.3 Surgical Indications and Contraindications

As recommended by Powell and Riley, the indications of surgery are as follows [1] (Tables 10.1 and 10.2):

Table 10.1 Powell and Riley indications for surgery

Indications of surgery	
1	AHI > 20
2	Oxygen saturation nadir <90%
3	Esophageal pressure more negative than −10 cm of H$_2$O
4	Cardiovascular problems [Arrhythmia/hypertension]
5	Neurobehavioral issues [Excessive daytime sleepiness]
6	Failure of medical management
7	Anatomical sites of obstruction

Table 10.2 Contraindications for OSA surgery

Contraindications of surgery	
1	Morbid obesity
2	Unstable cardiovascular disease
3	Severe pulmonary disease
4	Alcohol or drug abuse
5	Psychiatric instability
6	Unrealistic expectation

10.3.1   Surgeries for Snoring/ UARS/ OSA

- Nasal surgeries
- Palatal surgeries—Minimally invasive surgery/reshaping surgeries
- Tongue base surgeries—Minimally invasive tongue base surgeries/reshaping surgeries
- Hypopharyngeal surgery
- Maxillary mandibular advancement
- Hypoglossal nerve stimulation
- Tracheostomy
- Bariatric surgery.

10.3.1.1   Protocol for Surgery

OSAHS is associated with multiple levels of obstruction and hence to achieve a cure, a multi-level surgery may be needed.

It is necessary to understand that all the levels of obstruction must be addressed in an organized and a safe manner and hence Powell and Riley came up with a two-phase surgical protocol to target anatomical sites of obstruction.

This protocol was developed to minimalize the surgical procedures and avoid unnecessary surgery while alleviating patients' symptoms.

10.4   Powell–Riley Two-Phase Surgical Protocol: [2]

This protocol was directed toward treating specific anatomical sites of obstruction. They are divided into two phases. Phase 1 surgeries are conservative surgeries directed toward soft tissue of upper airway, while Phase 2 surgeries are more radical and considered when the patient does not alleviate of his symptoms after a phase 1 surgery. In very rare situations it may be necessary to perform phase 2 surgeries as an initial surgical procedure.

The list of Phase 1 and Phase 2 surgeries is given below (Table 10.3)

10.4.1   Surgical Procedures

10.4.1.1   Nasal Surgery

Nasal surgery is PIVOTAL and not PRIMARY in the management of OSA. Nasal airway contributes to two thirds of upper airway resistance and a compromise in the nasal airway will lead to SDB.

If nasal obstruction, snoring, and mouth breathing do not improve after medication or the patient is complaint to CPAP owing to a static obstruction in the nose, then a nasal surgery must be considered.

Isolated nasal surgery may help in compliance to CPAP and also help simple snorers or MILD OSA but when combined with other multilevel procedure it can cure even moderate to severe OSA [3].

Treatment of nasal obstruction has 3 potential goals:

Table 10.3 Powell–Riley two-phase surgical protocol

Phase 1 surgeries
Nasal surgery
Tonsillectomy
Uvulopalatopharyngoplasty [All palatal surgeries]
Tongue base surgeries
Mandibular osteotomy with genioglossus advancement
Hyoid myotomy and suspension
Temperature controlled radiofrequency reduction of turbinate, palate, and tongue base
Phase 2 surgeries
Maxillary mandibular advancement
Radiofrequency assisted reduction of tongue base

- Reduces nasal obstruction
- Reduces severity of SDB
- To facilitate compliance to CPAP.

Surgery for Nasal Valve (Figs. 10.1 and 10.2)
Nasal valve is the narrowest area of the nasal cavity which is bounded by septum medially, lower

border of upper lateral cartilage superiorly, and head of inferior turbinate laterally.

Any narrowing here causes nasal obstruction leading to mouth breathing and snoring.

Fig. 10.1 Surgical anatomy of internal nasal valve

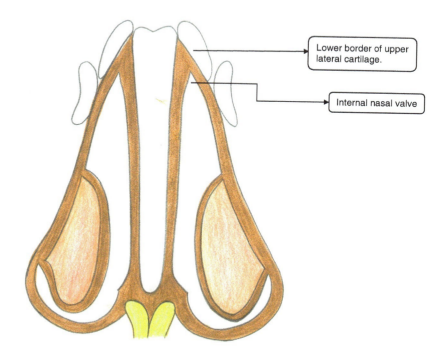

Lower border of upper lateral cartilage.

Internal nasal valve

Fig. 10.2 Nasal valve suspension

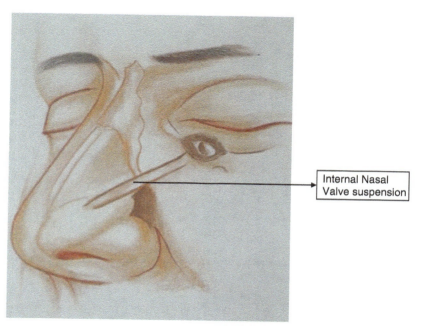

Internal Nasal Valve suspension

Radiofrequency/Coblation Reduction
of Inferior Turbinate (Figs. 10.3, 10.4 and 10.5)

Choice of Instruments

Reduction of inferior turbinate's can be
achieved with cold instruments or radiofrequency or Coblator, each technique having its
own advantage and disadvantage.

Patient Selection

Any patient with hypertrophic inferior turbinate
not responding to medical therapy and the turbinate is one of the causes of nasal obstruction [4].

Fig. 10.3 Radiofrequency
assisted reduction of inferior turbinate

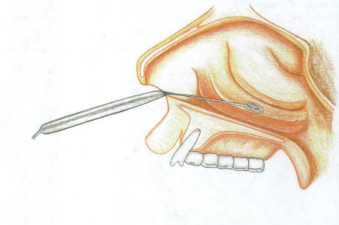

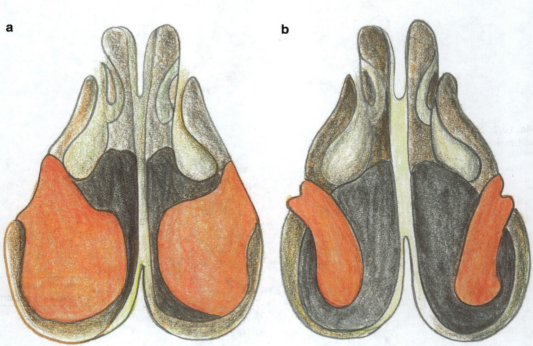

Fig. 10.4 (**a**) Prior to radiofrequency application; (**b**) Post radiofrequency application

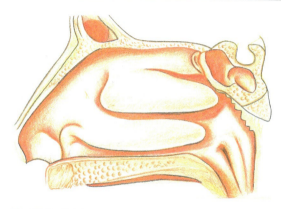

Fig. 10.5 Coblation inferior turbinate channeling

Septoplasty

It is a surgery aimed at correction of the nasal septum thus improving the nasal airway.

Candidates for Surgery

- All patients with DNS causing a compromise in the nasal airway on one side/both sides with chief complaints of nasal obstruction.
- xylometazoline test result is negative
- -those patients in whom rhinomanometry with pre and post xylometazoline are not encouraging are candidates for surgical correction.

Technique

This can be done endoscopically or in a classical way with the cold instruments or endoscopically.

Minor deviations or spur can be corrected endoscopically while a gross spur or deviations would need a conventional septoplasty approach.

10.4.1.2   Palatal Procedure

Minimally Invasive Procedure

Radiofrequency Assisted Uvulopalatoplasty (Fig. 10.6)
It is a radiofrequency assisted procedure that involves sequential reduction and reshaping of the tissues of uvula and palate.

Candidate Selection

- It is suitable for those patients with palatal snoring, with MILD OSAHS with excessive redundant tissue in the velopharyngeal area.
- The obstruction should be at the level of velum. Typically FTP 1 and 2 are ideal candidates.
- BMI less than 28 kg/m².

Procedure

This procedure can be performed under local anesthesia or general anesthesia. A monopolar radiofrequency probe is used for cutting the tissue.

The soft palate is primarily transected 1.0–1.5 cm bilaterally, parallel to the uvula and partial uvular resection is done with transversal resection of the distal 1–2 cm of the uvula from side to side by leaving intact mucosa on both [5].

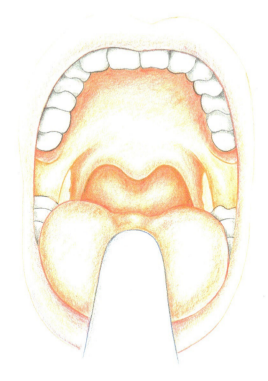

Fig. 10.6 Radiofrequency assisted uvulopalatoplasty

Contraindications
- Patients with small mouth or trismus
- Uncooperative patients with excessive gag reflex
- Submucosal cleft palate.

Complications
Stenosis at the level of palate/velum is one of the commonest complications associated with this procedure.

Apart from routine complications like bleeding and infection, there are chances of nasopharyngeal stenosis, palatal incompetence, and taste alteration, although rare in occurrence.

Partial Uvulectomy (Fig. 10.7)
It is a technique designed for those patients who are diagnosed with UARS.

Candidate Selection
Patients with UARS/elongated uvula touching the base of tongue and normal respiratory indices are ideal candidates [6].

Procedure
This procedure can be done under local anesthesia in an office-based setting or under general anesthesia as a part of other procedures. The length of the uvula measures from the base to the tip and the uvula may be amputated high or mid or low as shown in the diagram [6].

Instrumentation
A radiofrequency snare or coblation wand can be used for doing this procedure.

Complications
No major complications have been reported except pain, infection, dysphagia, vasovagal attacks and in rare situations palatal incompetence may occur.

Radiofrequency Assisted Palatal Stiffening Operation [Somnoplasty] (Fig. 10.8)
Majority of snoring is attributed to palatal flutter and techniques that stiffen palate are often considered in the treatment OSAHS.

Fig. 10.7 Partial
Uvulectomy

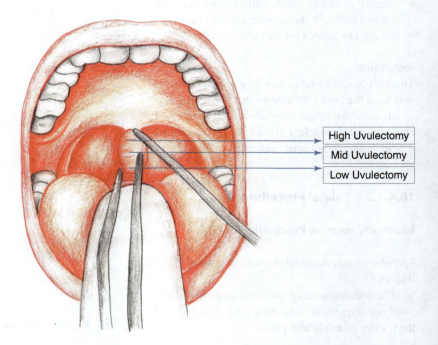

High Uvulectomy

Mid Uvulectomy

Low Uvulectomy

Candidate Selection

- Patients with MILD OSA
- Primary snorers [AHI<5]
- BMI<33
- Tonsil grade 1 and 2
- Patients with elongated uvula and excessive palatal mucosa.
- Patients with NO or minimal tongue base collapse.

Contraindications

- Nasal obstruction
- Distance between the tonsil is <2 cm
- Excessive palatal and pharyngeal redundant tissue
- Tongue base snoring
- FTP 3 or 4
- Retrognathia/TB hypertrophy/floppy epiglottis
- BMI >32
- Children.

Procedure

This procedure can be done under local anesthesia as an office-based procedure or can be done in general anesthesia in non-cooperative patient.

Points for insertion of radiofrequency probe [7]:

1. Midline between line 1 and 2.
2. Two lateral points midway between the uvula and the anterior pillar.

Various modifications are performed depending on patient's anatomy, the standard procedure is shown below.

Complications

No major complications are seen with this procedure except bleeding and scarring.

Modified Cautery-Assisted Palatal Stiffening Operation [Modified Capso]/ Anterior Palatoplasty (Fig. 10.9)

Palatal flutter is one of the commonest causes of snoring and techniques that stiffen the palate would yield a good result in reduction of the snoring.

Various techniques with variety of instruments were used to perform this procedure of stiffening of the palate.

The original cautery-assisted palatal stiffening operation (CAPSO) procedure was based on

Fig. 10.8 Somnoplasty

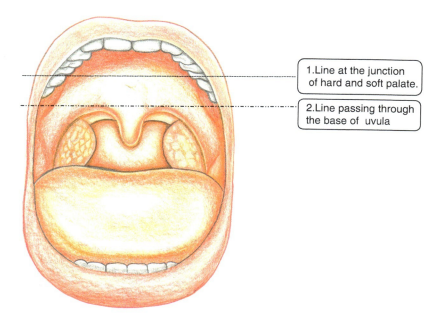

1. Line at the junction of hard and soft palate.

2. Line passing through the base of uvula

stripping a diamond-shaped area of mucosa off the soft palate and uvula, with the aid of cautery under local anesthesia but this procedure resulted in a scar on the anterior surface of the palate with tenting of the lateral pharyngeal walls. Hence a modification of this procedure was introduced by Pang et al where horizontal strip of mucosa was removed from the anterior surface of the palate and releasing incisions on the posterior soft palatal arches with a partial uvular trimming as needed. This procedure was named modified CAPSO or anterior palatoplasty [8].

Candidate Selection: [8]
• Patients who have palatal snoring/UARS/Mild OSA
• AHI <15 or AHI <5 but primary snorers
• Patient with age > 18 years
• BMI <33
• Tonsil grade 1 and 2
• Elongated uvula
• Minimum or no tongue base collapse.

Complications
Although rare, complications like bleeding, velopharyngeal insufficiency, fistula of the soft palate, and nasopharyngeal stenosis may occur [8].

Injection Snoreplasty (Fig. 10.10)
It is simple procedure aimed at injecting sclerosing agents into the palate for patients who are simple snorers.

The goal is to produce a superficial slough on the soft palate mucosa that is replaced by a scar tissue thus causing stiffening of the palate [9].

Candidate Selection
Patients who are primary snorers, suffering from socially bothersome snoring, UARS, and Mild OSA [9].

Sclerosing Agents: [9]
1. 3% sodium tetradecyl sulfate
2. 2% lidocaine with 98% dehydrated ethanol
3. Aethoxysklerol.

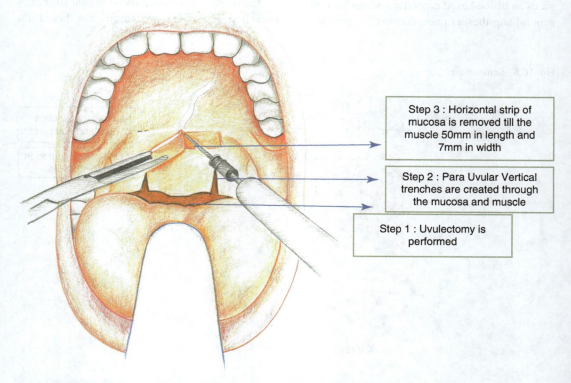

Step 3 : Horizontal strip of mucosa is removed till the muscle 50mm in length and 7mm in width

Step 2 : Para Uvular Vertical trenches are created through the mucosa and muscle

Step 1 : Uvulectomy is performed

Fig. 10.9 Modified cautery assisted uvulopalatoplasty operation/anterior palatoplasty

Procedure

A 0.5–2 ml submucosal injection is given with a 27gauge long needle into the soft palate, anterior to the hard palate and soft palate junction. It should not be given above the uvula as it causes swelling of the uvula and discomfort for the patient [9].

Complications

No major complications have been noted except ulceration and sloughing at the injection site [9].

Palatal Implants (Fig. 10.11)

In 2001, palatal implants were introduced to stiffen the soft palate. These are cylindrical implants made of polyethylene terephthalate.

The goal is to extend the hard palate into the soft palate and thus decrease the vibrations.

The advantage of this procedure is there is no resection or ablation of the tissue.

Patient Selection: [10]

- Patients without any morphological abnormality of the nose, nasopharynx, and hypopharynx are the candidates for isolated palatal implants.
- BMI<30
- Tonsils<grade 2
- Tongue position <grade 2.

If any of the following are present, then it is better to avoid a solitary implant procedure and combine it with other procedures as well. These include [10]

- Nasal obstruction
- Distance between tonsils is less than 2 cm
- Excessive palatal and pharyngeal mucosa
- Tongue base obstruction/hypertrophy with FTP 3 or 4
- Retrognathia
- Floppy epiglottis
- Obesity of 32 kg/m^2.

Procedure

It consists of a preloaded implant in the delivery tool.

Fig. 10.10 Injection snoreplasty

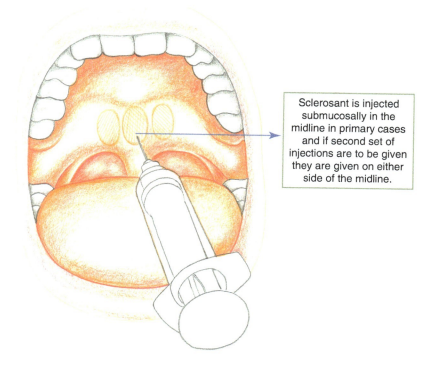

Sclerosant is injected submucosally in the midline in primary cases and if second set of injections are to be given they are given on either side of the midline.

The delivery tool is positioned at the junction of hard and soft palate in the midline. The needle has three markings on the tip. One indicating tip of the needle, second one indicating half insertion, and third one indicating full insertion of the implant. Once the implant is inserted then the plastic sleeve covering the tip of the needle must be removed [10].

Care must be taken to be always in the muscular layer [10].

Two lateral implants are inserted 2 mm lateral to the midline implant.

Additional two more implants may be inserted if it is deemed necessary.

Complications

Implant extrusion is one of the commonly associated complications in this procedure and hence should be avoided in patients who have under-gone an injection snoreplasty or coblation chan-neling of the palate or CAPSO because of prior tissue fibrosis, there is a higher risk of extrusion of the implant [10].

Barbed Pharyngoplasty/Barbed Snore Surgery [BSS]

To reduce the invasiveness of various surgical procedures, barbed pharyngoplasty was intro-duced. This technique requires the insertion of 3 sutures called as barbed sutures through the fibromuscular layer of the soft palate and then these sutures are tied around the posterior nasal spine and two pterygoid hamuli to obtain a stiff-ened soft palate which is capable of lifting and enlarging the oropharyngeal inlet and thus increasing the space across the palatopharyn-geus–retropalatal space [11].

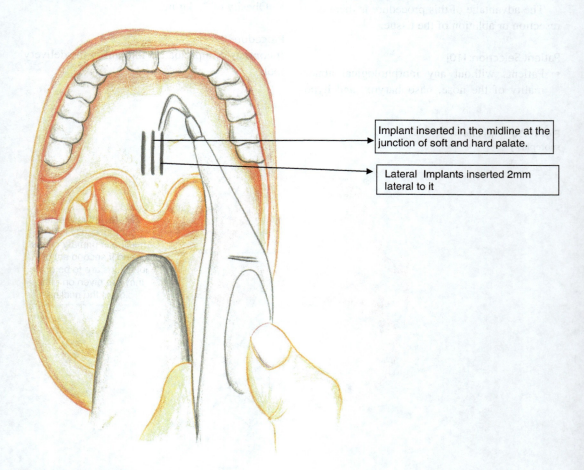

Implant inserted in the midline at the junction of soft and hard palate.

Lateral Implants inserted 2mm lateral to it

Fig. 10.11 Palatal implants

Properties of Barbed Sutures: [12]
- Sutures to be used only intratissue
- Knot free tissue closure sutures
- Bidirectional sutures
- Allow homogenous distribution of tensile forces thus producing an optimal scar and thereby the widening
- Most often reabsorbed by 180 days
- Commonly used is polydiaxone [PDO] (size 0 or 2-0, 36 cm × 36 cm or 40 × 40 cm configuration, on taper-pointed 36 or 26 mm semicircular needles).

Candidate Selection: [12]
- Mild to moderate OSA
- Simple snoring
- UARS
- Patients with retropalatal obstruction seen on DISE and having excessive bulk of palate and/or lateral pharyngeal wall.

Advantages: [12]
- Easy to learn
- Quick, safe, and effective
- Knotless absorbable suture technology
- Minimal mucosal and muscle resection.

Complications: [12]
- Tonsillar hemorrhage
- Infection
- Thread extrusion
- Granuloma formation
- Occasionally nasal regurgitation.

The various types of barbed surgery are classified below

Barbed Lateral Pharyngoplasty (Fig. 10.12)
Indications: [12]
- Mild to moderate OSAHS
- Thin, short, or submucosally bifid uvulopalatal complex
- In patients with velopharyngeal insufficiency which was primarily induced by previous resective surgery
- Any tonsil size grade 1–4

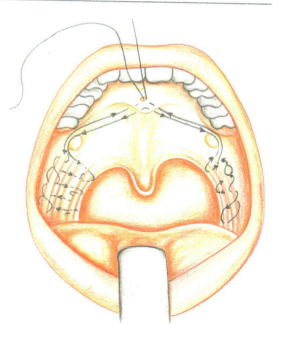

Fig. 10.12 Barbed lateral pharyngoplasty

- On examination with DISE there must be a *Laterolateral collapse* without any anteroposterior component.

Procedure

Barbed Anterior Palatoplasty (Fig. 10.13)
Indications: [12]
- This surgery is indicated in patients with mild OSAHS who have an enlarged elongated uvula with small tonsil [Grade 0 and 1]
- On examination with drug induced sleep endoscopy there must be an *Anteroposterior pattern of collapse.*

Barbed Roman Blind Technique (Fig. 10.14)
Indications: [12]
- Mild/moderate or severe OSAHS with functional uvulopalatal complex
- Tonsil size grade 1–grade 4
- On examination with DISE there must be a *Circular pattern of collapse.*

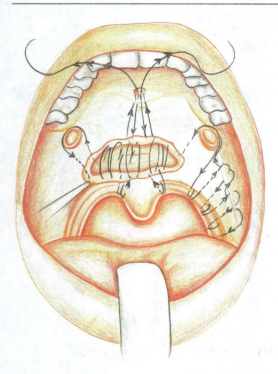

Fig. 10.13 Barbed anterior palatoplasty

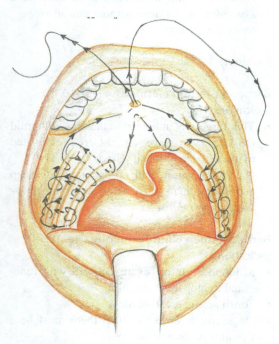

Fig. 10.14 Barbed roman blind technique

Barbed Alianza Technique: Alianza (BRBT + BAPh)
Indications: [12]
• Patients with snoring and mild to severe OSAHS
• Patients with thick uvula and palate with velopharyngeal patency and all tonsillar sizes
• On DISE: Circular pattern of collapse caused by the combination of the anteroposterior and laterolateral components.

This technique is a combination of barbed roman blind technique and barbed anterior pharyngoplasty. This technique leads to greater tensioning of the palate and pharyngeal walls [12].

10.4.1.3 Invasive Palatal Surgeries

Uvulopalatopharyngoplasty [UPPP]
(Figs. 10.15 and 10.16)
This was one of the most widely performed procedures but has been deemed obsolete now. This was first performed by Fujita in 1981 [13].

Candidate Selection (Table 10.4)

Procedure

UPPP with Fair Banks Modification
(Figs. 10.17 and 10.18)
Complications: [14]
• Airway obstruction due to airway edema
• Wound dehiscence and bleeding
• Transient velopharyngeal insufficiency
• Nasopharyngeal stenosis
• Change in voice.

Table 10.4 Indications of UPPP

Indications of UPPP [14]	
1	Posterior nasal spine to uvula distance >38 mm
2	Tonsil size grade 3 or grade 4
3	Posterior airway space >10 mm
4	Mandibular plane to hyoid distance <27 mm
5	Friedman tongue position 1 or 2
6	Absence of hypopharyngeal narrowing
7	Absence of morbid obesity
8	Absence of sagittal orientation of airway

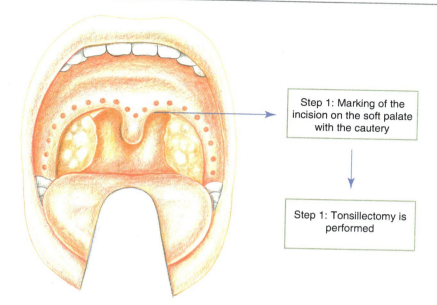

Fig. 10.15 Uvulopalatopharyngoplasty Step 1 and Step 2

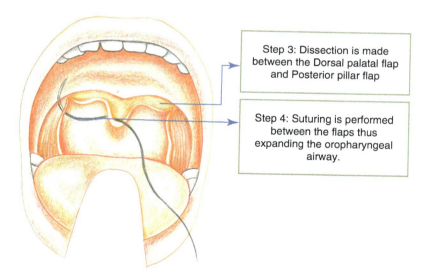

Fig. 10.16 Uvulopalatopharyngoplasty Step 3 and Step 4

Fig. 10.17 UPPP with Fairbanks modification Step 1 and Step 2

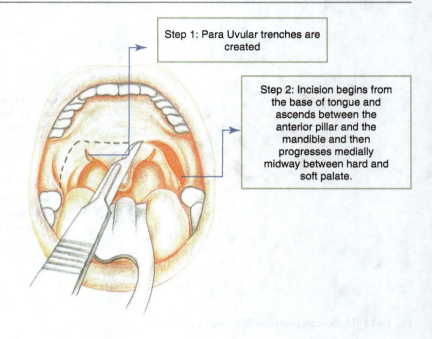

Step 1: Para Uvular trenches are created

Step 2: Incision begins from the base of tongue and ascends between the anterior pillar and the mandible and then progresses medially midway between hard and soft palate.

Fig. 10.18 UPPP with Fairbanks modification Step 3 and Step 4

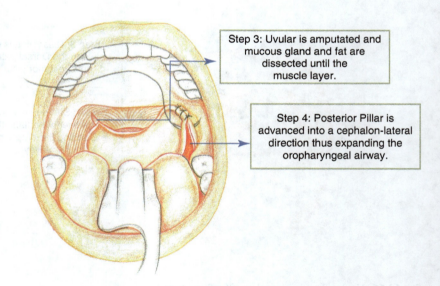

Step 3: Uvular is amputated and mucous gland and fat are dissected until the muscle layer.

Step 4: Posterior Pillar is advanced into a cephalon-lateral direction thus expanding the oropharyngeal airway.

Zetapalatopharyngoplasty [ZPP]
(Figs. 10.19, 10.20 and 10.21)

The goal of ZPP is to widen the space between the palate and the posterior pharyngeal wall, between palate and the tongue base and to either maintain or widen the dimensions of lateral pharyngeal wall [15].

This is achieved by two components

- A palatoplasty component—which involves removal of the mucosa of the palate and splitting the palate in midline
- Pharyngoplasty component—which involves tonsillectomy and pharyngeal closure.

Indications: [15]

- After a documented failure of CPAP trial
- Cases of previous tonsillectomy
- Cases of moderate to severe OSA with concentric narrowing at the level of soft palate on a DISE examination
- Friedman stage 2 and stage 3.

Contraindications: [15]

- A relative contraindication is when a patient is not willing for a CPAP trial and wants to undergo a surgery
- Friedman stage 1 and stage 4
- It is not a surgical option for patients with snoring only
- Craniofacial malformations.

Procedure
Principles: [15]

1. Tonsillectomy
2. Remove the soft palate mucosa
3. Splitting of the soft palate only in the midline
4. Cutting through the palatoglossus and palatopharyngeus to allow lateral expansion
5. Meticulous 2-layer closure.

Advantages: [15]
Despite aggressive palatal mucosal resection, the muscles of the soft palate are not excised thus eliminating the risk of permanent velopharyngeal insufficiency.

Disadvantages: [15]

- The procedure is irreversible
- There are no clear-cut landmarks or defined anatomical markings for the resection of the flap thus making surgeons judgement as final.

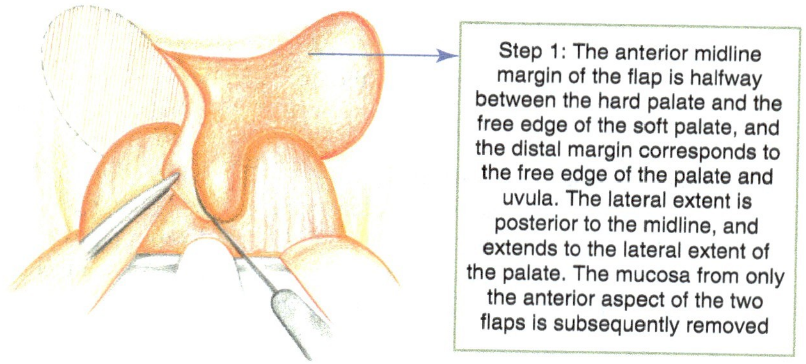

Fig. 10.19 Zetapalatoplasty Step 1

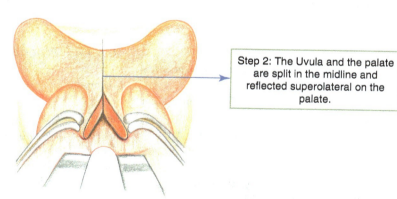

Step 1: The anterior midline margin of the flap is halfway between the hard palate and the free edge of the soft palate, and the distal margin corresponds to the free edge of the palate and uvula. The lateral extent is posterior to the midline, and extends to the lateral extent of the palate. The mucosa from only the anterior aspect of the two flaps is subsequently removed

Fig. 10.20 Zetapalatoplasty Step 2

Step 2: The Uvula and the palate are split in the midline and reflected superolateral on the palate.

Fig. 10.21 Zetapalatoplasty Step 3

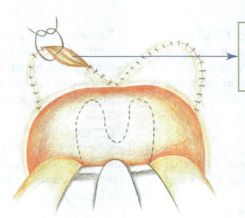

Step 3: Two layered closure of
the palatal flaps. The
submucosal layer is sutured
first with 2-0 Vicry followed by
the mucosal layer.

Complications: [15]
- Immediate post-operative pain and dysphagia
- Mild velopharyngeal insufficiency
- Foreign body sensation in throat.

Improvement after ZPP: [15]
- Subjective—symptom improvement
- Objective—On a polysomnography if there is a reduction in AHI below 20 or a 50% reduction in the AHI as compared to the pre-operative score.

What to do with Failure Cases of ZPP
Failure is defined as persistence of symptoms that demand additional treatment and when PSG score indicates a persistent disease [15].

The options for such patients are: [15]

1. CPAP therapy
2. DISE to identify the cause of persistent disease.

If there is a

- Retropalatal   obstruction—Advancement palatoplasty
- Retrolingual obstruction—Coblation tongue base reduction
- If all of the above fail, then a maxillary mandibular advancement.

Expansion Sphincter Pharyngoplasty
(Figs. 10.22, 10.23 and 10.24)
This procedure is aimed at addressing the lateral pharyngeal wall collapse in patients with OSA.

Candidate Selection: [16]
- Patients with retropalatal obstruction and lateral collapse
- Small tonsil size grade 1/2
- BMI <30
- Friedman stage 2 and 3 who have failed CPAP.

Procedure
Principle: [16]
1. Isolate the palatopharyngeus muscle and rotate it superolaterally in order to create a lateral wall tension and remove the trunk of lateral pharyngeal wall.
2. Keep a part of the palatopharyngeus muscle fibrous attachment to the superior constrictor.

Complications: [16]
- Infection and bleeding
- Fistula of soft palate.

10.4.1.4 Tongue Base Surgeries

Minimally Invasive Tongue Base Surgeries

Radiofrequency Assisted Reduction of Tongue Base Reduction (Fig. 10.25)
If tongue base obstruction is identified on evaluation, then this has to be addressed. Radiofrequency assisted reduction of tongue base works by using a 460 KHz, by a high-frequency alternating current flow into the tissue resulting in protein coagulation and necrosis [17].

Fig. 10.22 Expansion sphincter pharyngoplasty Step 1

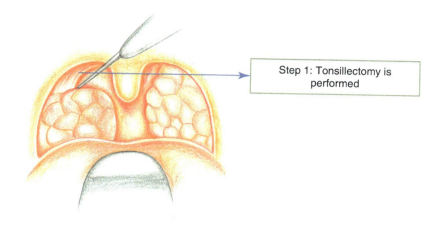

Step 1: Tonsillectomy is performed

Fig. 10.23 Expansion sphincter pharyngoplasty Step 2 and Step 3

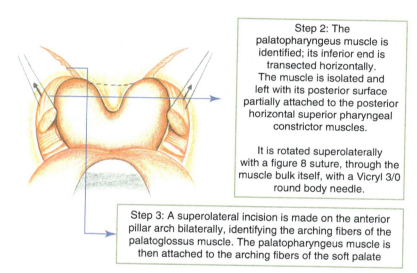

Step 2: The palatopharyngeus muscle is identified; its inferior end is transected horizontally. The muscle is isolated and left with its posterior surface partially attached to the posterior horizontal superior pharyngeal constrictor muscles.

It is rotated superolaterally with a figure 8 suture, through the muscle bulk itself, with a Vicryl 3/0 round body needle.

Step 3: A superolateral incision is made on the anterior pillar arch bilaterally, identifying the arching fibers of the palatoglossus muscle. The palatopharyngeus muscle is then attached to the arching fibers of the soft palate

Fig. 10.24 Expansion sphincter pharyngoplasty Step 4

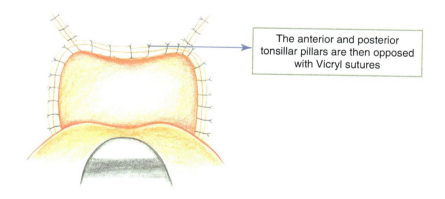

The anterior and posterior tonsillar pillars are then opposed with Vicryl sutures

This is followed by chronic inflammation, fibrosis, and scarring resulting in reduction in the tissue volume [17].

It must be understood that multiple procedures may be required to get adequate outcome.

Candidate Selection: [17]

Patients in whom tongue base collapse has been documented on preoperative evaluation.

Procedure

Probe

The radiofrequency probe is designed in such a way that it has a proximal end which is insulated and protects the superficial mucosa and musculature while the distal end is non-insulated which generates a target tissue temperature of 85°C [17].

Technique
Complications: [17]

- Tongue ulcerations and abscess formation
- Upper airway obstruction—either due to tongue hematoma or abscess or edema
- Hypoglossal nerve injury

- Temporary and permanent difficulty in swallowing
- Alterations in the taste.

Coblation Channeling of Tongue/Coblation Midline Glossectomy (Figs. 10.26 and 10.27)

This procedure aims at resecting the midline of the tongue with the help of Coblator and endoscopic guidance.

The goal is to reduce the tissue at the base of tongue and thus increase airway way space in the retrolingual area.

A preoperative ultrasonography is done to identify the course of lingual vessels.

It is very important to map the course of lingual artery with ultrasonography to prevent injury to it. Intraoperative Doppler may be used to confirm the location of the same [18].

Candidate Selection [18]

- Patients older than 18 years of age
- Patients with symptoms of OSA, AHI >15, and have either failed/refused a CPAP trial
- FTP-III/IV

Fig. 10.25 Radiofrequency assisted tongue base reduction

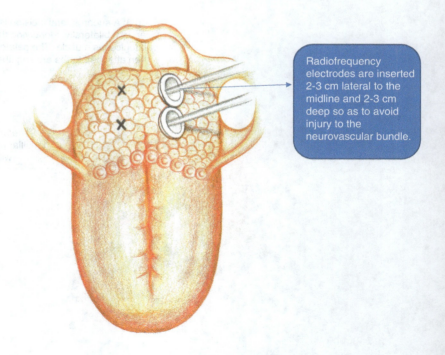

Radiofrequency electrodes are inserted 2-3 cm lateral to the midline and 2-3 cm deep so as to avoid injury to the neurovascular bundle.

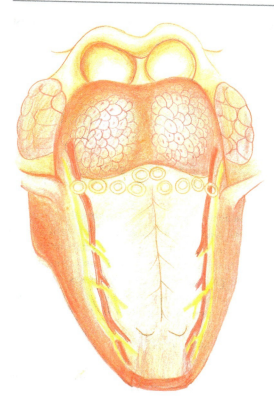

- Retrolingual obstruction identified on fiberoptic laryngopharyngoscopy with Mueller's maneuver and end expiratory tongue position or drug induced sleep endoscopy
- Body mass index <40 kg/m².

Contraindications: [18]
- Patients with trismus.

Procedure: [18]
The procedure is done under general anesthesia with nasotracheal intubation or orotracheal intubation.

Complications: [18]
- Bleeding from the lingual artery is one of the commonly anticipated complications
- Infection
- Pain and dysphagia
- Tongue edema leading to airway obstruction
- Hypoglossal nerve weakness.

Fig. 10.26 Lingual artery and lingual nerve

Fig. 10.27 Coblation Midline Glossectomy

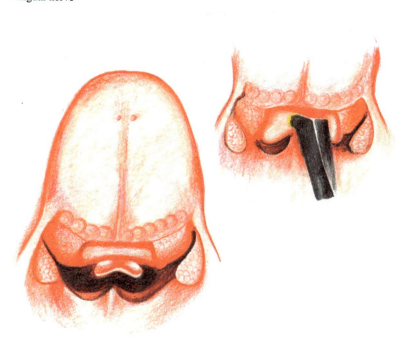

Tongue Base Stabilization (Fig. 10.28)

In patients with collapsed retrolingual space, stabilizing the tongue and the lower pharynx may effectively treat sleep-disordered breathing.

Candidate Selection

• It is ideal for patients who have decreased retrolingual space from sitting to supine position as evidenced by FLPscopy.

It is contraindicated in patients with macroglossia, abnormal mandibular bone, poor oral hygiene, and periodontal diseases [19].

Procedure

Complications: [19]

• Injury to neurovascular bundle—osteomyelitis
• Damage to dental structures and ducts of salivary gland mainly the Wharton's duct.

Lingual Tonsillectomy

It is important to differentiate pathology of base of tongue from lingual tonsil hypertrophy. If the lingual tonsils are >10 mm in diameter and abutting the posterior border of tongue and posterior pharyngeal wall, then they are considered enlarged [20].

A lingual tonsil must be differentiated from muscular tongue base and tumors. This can be done by performing a preoperative contrast enhanced MRI which will help in differentiating the same [20].

Procedure: [20]

The patient is placed in rose position and with the help of Evac70 Coblator wand, the lingual tissue from the base of tongue is resected.

Invasive Tongue Base Surgery

Genioglossus Advancement (Figs. 10.29 and 10.30)

This is a surgery aimed at enlarging the hypopharyngeal area. In this surgery a rectangular osteotomy is performed without interrupting the lower margin of mandible and this segment [21].

This procedure basically increases the tension of the muscle in order to compensate for the collapse of tongue during sleep.

Candidate Selection: [21]

• Documented hypopharyngeal obstruction based on physical examination and cephalometry
• Fujita type II (retropalatal and retrolingual) or type III (retrolingual) abnormality with evidence of moderate to severe obstructive sleep apnea
• Patients who have failed palatal surgery
• As a part of multilevel surgery.

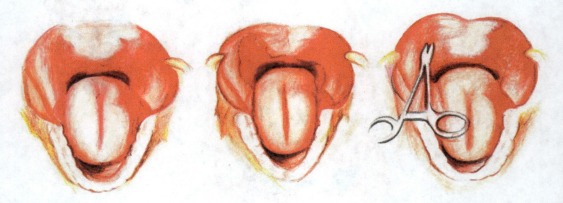

Fig. 10.28 Tongue base stabilization

Procedure

Complications: [21]
- Mandibular fractures
- Floor of the mouth hematoma
- Edema of tongue and floor of mouth
- Paresthesia of lower teeth
- Wound dehiscence and infection
- Detachment of muscle and extrusion of osteo-synthesis material.

TORS [Transoral Robotic Surgery]

This procedure involves robotic assisted resection of a part of base of tongue from the foramen cecum to the valleculae.

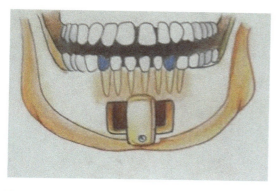

Fig. 10.29 Genioglossus Advancement Step 1

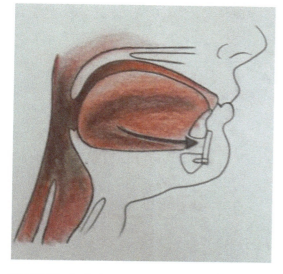

Fig. 10.30 Genioglossus Advancement Step 2

Candidate Selection: [22]
- Moderate to severe OSA with symptoms
- The best candidates for TORS are those patients with localized, low (within the epiglottic valleculas area), lymphoid tongue base obstruction.

Contraindications: [22]
- Unstable cardiovascular disease, neuromuscular disease, need for anticoagulation, significant psychological instability
- Local contraindications to the procedure include micrognathia and macroglossia (with high modified Mallampati–Friedman scores).

Instrumentation: [22]
- The 12-mm, 30-degree 3-D scope (upward facing) is used
- Two robotic 5-mm Endo Wrist devices are used for each patient
- Maryland dissector for grasping and dissecting tissues
- Monopolar cautery with a spatula tip for dissection and coagulation.

Surgical Team

Primary and secondary surgeon with bedside technician.

Procedure: [22]

Exposure robot is docked.

Right and left lingual tonsillectomy is done and the residual obstruction to the tongue base is evaluated and further resection is done with precaution to avoid trauma to the lingual vessels.

Postoperative Care and Complications: [22]
- In view of airway edema that could occur postoperatively delayed extubation or a temporary tracheostomy may be performed
- Feeding is provided with nasogastric tube
- Other delayed complications include teeth injury, voice change, and dysgeusia.

Supraglottoplasty (SGP) (Fig. 10.31)

This technique is used in conditions where there is a primary or secondary epiglottic collapse. It can be performed as an isolated procedure or as a part of TORS.

The role of SGP is to prevent the inward collapse of the floppy epiglottis and/or redundant supraglottic tissue [22].

Indications: [22]
Moderate to severe OSA with EDS.

Contraindications: [22]
Patients who can be successfully managed with conservative surgery Retrognathia

Neck stiffness and inter-incisor distance is less than 1.5 cm.

Procedure: [22]
The aryepiglottic fold is incised so that the epiglottis is released and moves away from the glottic inlet toward the tongue base.

Steps:

- Vertical midline suprahyoid epiglottic split
- Horizontal epiglottic resection
- The horizontal transection should be above the level of pharyngoepiglottic fold to minimize aspiration and avoid bleeding from branches of superior laryngeal vessels.

The safer technique for avoiding postoperative edema and for avoiding damage to the superior laryngeal vascular bundle is the "V-shape" epiglottoplasty. A V-shape wedge is removed from the central and superior area of the epiglottis [22].

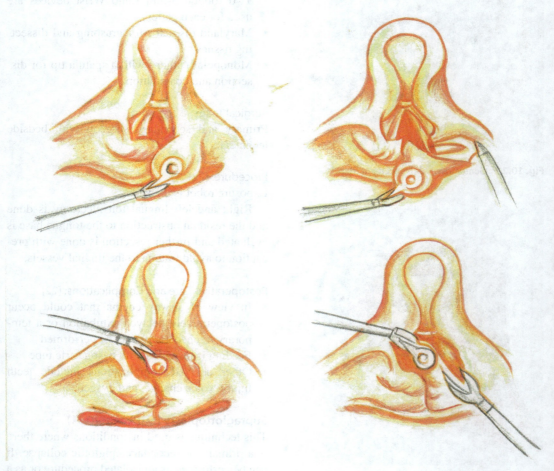

Fig. 10.31 Supraglottoplasty

Hyoid Suspension (Fig. 10.32)

It is a procedure aimed at increasing the retrolingual airway space.

Hyoid suspension is often performed in combination with genioglossus advancement (GA) and followed by maxillomandibular osteotomy (MMO) as phased surgery in case of failure [23].

It can be done as an isolated procedure as well.

Candidate Selection: [23]

- Moderate to severe OSA with retroglossal collapse noted on clinical examination and drug induced sleep endoscopy
- Friedman stage 2 and 3
- Small tonsil and normal uvula without a floppy epiglottis or a palatal stenosis after UPPP.

Surgical Procedure: [23]

Principle

- Stabilization of the hyoid bone inferiorly by attachment to superior border of thyroid cartilage
- Anterior movement of the hyoid complex increases the posterior airway space and neutralizes obstruction at the tongue base.

Procedure

- Inferior attachment of the strap muscles is cut from hyoid
- 2+2 permanent sutures are placed between the hyoid and superior border of thyroid cartilage on either side.

Complications: [23]

- Tongue hematoma
- Swallowing and speech problems.

Epiglottis Management

Technique 1: Epiglottopexy with or without lingual tonsillectomy [24]. Technique 2: Laser epiglottectomy [24].

Indication

Epiglottic collapse.

Instruments

1. Coblation
2. Diathermy with laparoscopy scissors
3. Harmonic scalpel
4. Radiofrequency.

Procedure

- Nasal intubation
- Rose position

Fig. 10.32 Hyoid suspension

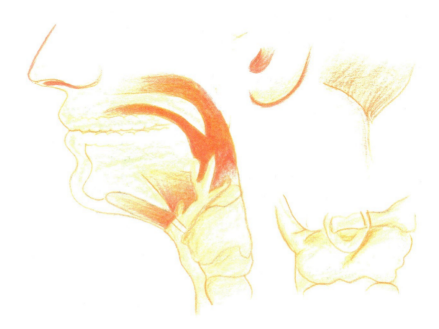

- Small tongue blade/Boyle Davis gag
- Tongue suture to pull it out
- 0° or 30° endoscope
- MLS instruments
- Insulated suction diathermy.

Complications
1. Bleeding
2. Aspiration.

Maxillary Mandibular Advancement
This surgery achieves enlargement of the pharyngeal and the hypopharyngeal airway by physically expanding the skeletal framework.

This is a procedure that involves advancement of maxilla and mandible via Le Fort 1 and sagittal split osteotomies, respectively.

It is a global airway procedure for OSA. With the advancement of maxilla and mandible there is advancement of soft palate, tongue base, and hyoid bone with associated increase in velopharyngeal and hypopharyngeal airway without direct manipulation of pharyngeal tissues.

Candidate Selection
There is no final consensus if this surgery should be the initial surgical treatment or reserved as a LAST RESORT in patients in whom the other treatment modalities have failed.

This surgery should be considered in patients who have a "DISPROPORTIONATE" maxillofacial feature.

Surgical decision is usually based on surgeon's preference, experience, patients airway and skeletal anatomy, severity of OSAS, and the patients desire.

Procedure [25]
- Prior to surgery, a methylmethacrylate occlusal splint and preformed arch bars are fabricated for the alignment of the mobilized dental segments during surgery
- Extraction of both bicuspids
- A horizontal subapical osteotomy is made about 5 mm below the teeth apices
- Le Fort I osteotomy and down-fracturing of the maxilla

- A vertical interdental osteotomy is carried out between the sockets. Completion of the transpalatal osteotomies bilaterally will free the premaxilla
- The maxilla and the mandible are advanced 10 mm
- Grafting and fixation done
- Confirm segments position and implant placement
- The occlusal splint is left in situ for stabilization of the occlusion, and intermaxillary fixation is left in place for up to 6 weeks.

Post-operative Management
1. Airway control
2. Hemodynamic stability
3. Prevention of ischemia to bone
4. Prevention of wound infection
5. Antihypertensive
6. Narcotic analgesic
7. Nasal decongestants
8. Oral and nasal toilet
9. IV steroids
10. IV antibiotics

Complications: [25]
1. Aseptic necrosis of maxilla and mandible
2. Skeletal fixation
3. Malocclusion [Dental]
4. Velopharyngeal insufficiency
5. Paraesthesia—Paraesthesia of upper and lower lips recovers between 6 to 12 months
6. Aspiration
7. Implant related problem.

Tracheostomy
Kuhlo in 1968 described tracheostomy for OSA. Feetward described "Skin lined flap tracheostomy" to overcome in obese patients with OSA. Goal is to create a permanent stoma of 8–10 mm [26].

Candidate Selection
For patients who are intolerant of mechanical measures or fail upper airway surgery and continue to have severe symptoms or physiologic changes related to obstructive sleep apnea, flap tracheostomy is a reasonable alternative [26].

Procedure [26]

- A horizontally designed "H" with extension of the flaps superiorly and inferiorly and laterally
- Lipectomy
- The vertical "H" incision used to incise the trachea transversally at tracheal ring three, with an inferior flap slightly longer than the superior
- Suturing of skin to trachea
- Once complete healing has occurred and the patient is prepared to occlude the tracheostomy tube while active and awake, and to open the lumen only for sleep
- Custom-made stoma closure by orthodontist or Montgomery tracheal cannula.

Complications

1. Dehiscence and necrosis of flap, creating a granulating wound
2. Malodorous drainage
3. Bleeding during tracheostomy tube change or cleaning
4. Stomal stenosis.

Speech Ready Long-Term Tube-Free Tracheostomy

Indication [27]

1. RDI > 50
2. $SpO_2 < 60$
3. Cor pulmonale
4. Cardiac dysrhythmias
5. Epileptic experiencing seizures in apnea.

Technique [27]

- Best performed in patients without previous tracheostomy
- Omega shaped incision located 1 cm above clavicles extending beyond sternocleidomastoid laterally
- Dome of omega reaches up to cricoid bone
- Separate the strap muscles in the midline
- Isthmus of thyroid divided
- Thyroid lobes dissected anterolaterally from trachea and are sutured to sternal tendon of sternocleidomastoid

- Superiorly based flap in anterior tracheal wall at the level of 2nd and 3rd rings or 3rd and 4th rings
- Margins of skin flap are brought together and sutured to tracheal opening.

Few cases require supplementary sling procedure after several months. Here superiorly based SCM muscle flap is tunneled and sutured to the inferiorly based SCM muscle flap inferior to the stoma. This helps in voluntary closure of stoma.

LTTF speech ready tracheostomy is the gold standard for management of severe chronic upper airway obstruction [27].

Advantages [27]

1. Aspiration prevented
2. Normal laryngeal reflex
3. Cough present
4. Will be able to smell.

Disadvantages of Tube Dependent Techniques

1. Granulations
2. Posterior wall stenosis
3. Erosion of upper trachea
4. Infection
5. Increased secretions.

Hypoglossal Nerve Stimulation

The primary muscles involved in maintaining airway patency are the intrinsic and extrinsic muscles of the tongue, which are innervated by the HGN.

During sleep, decreased tonic stimulation of the hypoglossal motor nucleus contributes to a loss of tonicity in muscle fibers, which in turn contributes to upper airway collapse in those patients who are predisposed to OSA due to constrictive anatomy and/or increased extraluminal pressure [28].

Indications

HNS therapy is currently indicated for moderate to severe OSA patients who are CPAP-intolerant, have a body mass index <32, apnea–hypopnea index <50, and without a concentric pattern of upper airway collapse on sleep endoscopy [28].

Contraindications [28]

1. BMI > 32 kg/m^2
2. Concentric pattern of upper airway collapse
3. More than 25% of central sleep apneas
4. Positional OSA (>50% reduction in AHI between supine and non-supine positions)
5. Tonsil size greater than type 2
6. Tongue malformations; alteration of tongue motor activity
7. Marked salivation disorders
8. Neuromuscular disease
9. Hypoglossal nerve palsy
10. Active psychiatric disease; other non-respiratory sleep disorders
11. Pregnancy
12. Major systemic disorder
13. Requirement of magnetic resonance imaging.

Procedure [28]

- A 5 cm incision is made one finger breadth below the mandibular margin, anteriorly up to midline and posteriorly to the submandibular gland
- Dissection is done to identify the main trunk of hypoglossal nerve which is traced anteriorly
- The medial and lateral branches are identified and confirmed using a nerve integrity monitoring system (NIM, Medtronic Xome®)
- The electrode cuff is wrapped around the medial branches in Inspire II device, while in the ImThera Medical Inc. the electrode cuff is rolled under and around the main trunk of the nerve
- The pleural pressure sensing lead is placed through a horizontal incision that is made at the right fourth or fifth intercostal space lateral to the nipple line
- A pocket is tunneled postero-anteriorly between external and internal intercostal muscle layers where the sensing lead faces pleura
- The implantable pulse generator (IPG) connects the nerve stimulation cuff and the pleural sensing electrode
- A subcutaneous pectoral pocket is created 2–5 cm inferior to the right clavicle and medial

to the deltopectoral groove. Inferiorly the pocket is extended subcutaneously to the pleural sensing electrode. Superiorly, a subplatysmal tunnel is created to the hypoglossal nerve stimulation cuff, and the lead passed downwards and connected to (IPG).

Stimulation Protocol [28]

The Inspire II system is activated 4 weeks post-implantation, and the stimulation is given between end expiration through the inspiratory period to minimize neuromuscular fatigue. Titration is performed at 1, 2, and 4 months post-implantation.

The ImThera medical system is activated in seated awake patients 3 to 4 weeks after surgery. Electrodes are stimulated cyclically in a pattern independent of the respiratory cycle and titrations performed at 1 and 12 months post-implantation.

Complications [28]

1. Numbness/pain at incision site
2. Hematoma/seroma
3. Malfunction of devise
4. Dislodgement of the stimulation lead cuff
5. Soreness of tongue
6. Temporary weakness of tongue.

References

1. Powell NB, Riley RW. Surgical management for obstructive sleep- disordered breathing. In: Principles and practice of sleep medicine. 5th ed. Philadelphia: Elsevier; 2010. p. 1250–65.
2. Powell NB. Contemporary surgery for obstructive sleep apnea syndrome. Clin Exp Otorhinolaryngol [Internet]. 2009 Sep;2(3):107–14. [cited 2021 Feb 27]. Available from: https://www.ncbi.nlm.nih.gov/pmc/articles/PMC2751873/.
3. Sethukumar P, Kotecha B. Tailoring surgical interventions to treat obstructive sleep apnoea: One size does not fit all. Breathe [Internet]. 2018 Sep 1;14(3):e84–93. [cited 2021 Feb 27]. Available from: https://www.ncbi.nlm.nih.gov/pmc/articles/PMC6196320/.
4. Li KK. Radiofrequency volumetric reduction for hypertrophic turbinate. In: Friedman M, editor. Snoring and sleep apnea. Philadelphia: Saunders Elsevier; 2009. p. 138–42.

5. Lim DJ, Kang SH, Kim BH, Kim HG. Treatment of primary snoring using radiofrequency-assisted uvulopalatoplasty. Eur Arch Oto-Rhino-Laryngology [Internet]. 2007 Jul 9;264(7):761–7. [cited 2021 Feb 28]. Available from: https://link.springer.com/article/10.1007/s00405-007-0252-x.

6. Newman J. Snare uvulectomy for upper airway resistance. In: Friedman M, editor. Sleep apnea and snoring. Philadelphia: Saunders Elsevier; 2009. p. 154–8.

7. Kezirian EJ. Radiofrequency of the palate. In: Rhinologic and sleep apnea surgical techniques [Internet]. Berlin: Springer; 2007. p. 303–8. [cited 2021 Feb 28]. Available from: https://link.springer.com/chapter/10.1007/978-3-540-34020-1_31.

8. Pang KP, Teris DJ. Cautery assisted palatal stiffening operation. In: Friedman M, editor. Snoring and sleep apnea. Philadelphia: Saunders Elsevier; 2009. p. 159–14.

9. Brietzke SE, Mair EA. Injection snoreplasty. In: Friedman M, editor. Sleep apnea and snoring. Philadelphia: Saunders Elsevier; 2009. p. 165–8.

10. Maurer JT. Palatal implants for primary snoring. In: Friedman M, editor. Sleep Apnea and Snoring [Internet]. Philadelphia: Elsevier; 2020. p. 177–83. Available from: https://linkinghub.elsevier.com/retrieve/pii/B9780323443395000316.

11. Mantovani M, Torretta S, TaSSone G. The "Barbed Roman Blinds" technique: a step forward La tecnica delle tende a pacchetto con "barbed suture": un passo in avanti. Acta Otorhinolaryngol Ital. 2013;33(2):128.

12. Mantovani M, Pignataro L. Barbed Snore Surgery (BSS). In: Friedman M, editor. Sleep apnea and snoring: surgical and non-surgical therapy. 2nd ed. Philadelphia: Elsevier; 2019. p. 235–9.

13. Fujita S, Conway W, Zorick F, Roth T. Surgical correction of anatomic abnormalities in obstructive sleep apnea syndrome: Uvulopalatopharyngoplasty. Otolaryngol – Head Neck Surg [Internet]. 1981 Nov 11;89(6):923–34. [cited 2021 Mar 7]. Available from: http://journals.sagepub.com/doi/10.1177/019459988108900609.

14. Katsantonis GP. Uvulopalatopharyngoplasty. In: Friedman M, editor. Sleep apnea and snoring. Philadelphia: Saunders Elsevier; 2009. p. 176–83.

15. Friedman M, Schalch P. Zetapalatopharyngoplasty (ZPP). In: Friedman M, editor. Sleep apnea and snoring. Philadelphia: Saunders Elsevier; 2009. p. 201–5.

16. Pang KP, Woodson BT. Expansion sphincter pharyngoplasty. In: Friedman M, editor. Sleep apnea and snoring. Philadelphia: Saunders Elsevier; 2009. p. 224–6.

17. Troell RJ. Radiofrequency tongue base reduction in sleep-disordered breathing. In: Friedman M, editor. Sleep apnea and snoring. Philadelphia: Elsevier; 2009. p. 243–7.

18. Lin HC, Friedman M. Endoscopic coblator open tongue base resection for obstructive sleep apnea. In: Friedman M, editor. Sleep apnea and snoring: surgical and non-surgical therapy. 2nd ed. Philadelphia: Elsevier; 2019. p. 257–61.

19. Tucker WB. A minimally invasive technique for tongue base stabilization. In: Friedman M, editor. Sleep apnea and snoring. Philadelphia: Elsevier; 2009. p. 258–64.

20. Michaelson PG, Mair EA. Endoscopic coblation lingual tonsillectomy. In: Friedman M, editor. Sleep apnea and snoring: surgical and non-surgical therapy. 2nd ed. Philadelphia: Elsevier; 2019. p. 267–9.

21. Li KK. Genioglossus advancement in sleep apnea surgery. In: Friedman M, editor. Sleep apnea and snoring. Philadelphia: Elsevier; 2009. p. 301–4.

22. Vicini C, Montevecchi F, Meccariello G. Transoral Robotic Surgery (TORS) for OSA. In: Friedman M, editor. Sleep apnea and snoring: surgical and non-surgical therapy. 2nd ed. Philadelphia: Elsevier; 2019. p. 315–8.

23. Benoist L, Ravesloot MJL, Maanen JP, Vries N. Hyoid suspension as the only procedure. In: Friedman M, editor. Sleep apnea and snoring: surgical and non-surgical therapy. 2nd ed. Philadelphia: Elsevier; 2019. p. 305–10.

24. Thaler ER. Management of the epiglottis. In: Friedman M, editor. Sleep apnea and snoring: surgical and non-surgical therapy. 2nd ed. Philadelphia: Elsevier; 2019. p. 311–4.

25. Hong Goh Y, Mark WT, Wah IH. Modified maxillomandibular advancement technique. In: Friedman M, editor. Sleep apnea and snoring. Philadelphia: Elsevier; 2009. p. 334–8.

26. Maisel RH. Tracheostomy for sleep apnea. In: Friedman M, editor. Sleep apnea and snoring. Philadelphia: Elsevier; 2009. p. 343–8.

27. Eliachar I, Akst LM, Lorenz RR. Speech-ready, long-termtube-free tracheostomy for obstructive sleep apnea. In: Friedman M, editor. Sleep apnea and snoring. Philadelphia: Elsevier; 2009. p. 349–60.

28. Sasidharan J, Vardhan H, Bhargava A, Gupta A. Hypoglossal nerve stimulation for obstructive sleep apnea: a novel surgical approach (A review of literature). Indian J Sleep Med [Internet]. 2018 Dec;13(4):67–70. [cited 2021 Mar 14]. Available from: https://www.ijsm.in/doi/10.5005/jp-journals-10069-0029.

Perioperative and Postoperative Considerations in Management of Patients with OSA

Obstructive sleep apnea (OSA) presents a major challenge to anesthetists. It is very important to have a proper preoperative evaluation, intraoperative management, postoperative care, and pain management in patients with OSA.

These patients are likely to have several co-morbidities which could possibly result in adverse outcomes. The effects of sedatives, analgesics, and anesthetics can worsen OSA by several mechanisms and there is an increased risk of anesthetic and postoperative complications.

11.1 Preoperative Consideration

Patients with OSA should be screened well prior to surgery in order to decide the anesthetic plan.

ASA guidelines recommend screening for symptoms like snoring, sudden awakening from sleep with a choking sensation, witnessed apnea by a bed partner, headaches, and daytime somnolence.

A prior airway assessment and physical examination must be conducted to assess the risks of intubation.

Polysomnography should be a routine preoperative investigation in all surgical patients who have two or more major symptoms of OSA.

The results of the sleep study in terms of showing mild, moderate, or severe disease should be used to determine the anesthetic management.

If the patient is suspected to have OSA and sleep studies are not available or if the surgery is an emergency, patients should be treated as though they have moderate sleep apnea.

Anesthetic management should be carefully planned in consultation with the surgeon.

Anesthetic drugs can greatly influence the outcomes in patients with co-morbidities and in those who already have a dysfunctional respiratory system.

It is advisable to use local anesthesia over general anesthesia (GA) whenever possible.

If general anesthesia is the only option, controlled ventilation with endotracheal intubation should be done. Endotracheal intubation is associated with a higher propensity for difficult intubation in obese patients as compared to the normal subjects.

Obesity, a short thick neck and excess pharyngeal tissue deposits in the lateral pharyngeal walls are causative factors for difficult intubation (Table 11.1). The Preoperative, Intraoperative and postoperative checklists are mentioned in Tables 11.1, 11.2, and 11.3.

D. S. Deenadayal, V. Bommakanti, *Management of Snoring and Obstructive Sleep Apnea*, https://doi.org/10.1007/978-981-16-6620-9_11

Table 11.1 Preoperative checklist for OSA

Preoperative check list	
1.	Anthropometric data like BMI/neck circumference/ hyomental distance
2.	Complete ENT examination
3.	Polysomnography
4.	DISE
5.	Cardiovascular, respiratory, and endocrinological evaluation
6.	Mallampati scoring

Table 11.2 Intraoperative considerations

Intraoperative considerations	
1.	Minimize surgical stress
2.	Reduce the duration of surgery
3.	Consider LA to GA
4.	Anticipate difficult intubation
5.	Consider awake intubation in a semi-upright position

Table 11.3 Postoperative considerations

Postoperative considerations	
1.	Minimize the use of opioids and sedation
2.	Consider the use of acetaminophen/NSAIDs
3.	Continuous monitoring of oxygen
4.	Postoperative PAP therapy
5.	Follow up

11.2 Intraoperative

11.2.1 Drugs and Monitoring

Various anesthetic drugs such as thiopentone, propofol, opioids, benzodiazepines, and nitrous oxide are known to reduce the tone of the pharyngeal musculature and cause airway collapse. Hence, these drugs should be avoided during surgery.

It is also better to avoid large doses of longer acting drugs, especially neuromuscular blocking agents. Shorter acting drugs are preferred as they return rapidly to baseline respiratory function. Opioids should be used judiciously.

No special monitoring is necessary but routine monitoring of heart rate, respiratory rate, and blood pressure should be done.

11.3 Intubation Technique

The anesthetist needs to be prepared for a difficult airway and the necessary equipment for the same should be available beforehand.

Orotracheal tubes in various sizes, gum elastic bougie as well as a McCoy laryngoscope and a laryngeal mask airway are necessary.

An algorithm should be decided prior to the procedure.

The decision to intubate, whether when the patient is awake or anesthetized, needs to be taken by the anesthetist depending on the individual patient's airway difficulty. This decision should be taken after a complete preoperative airway evaluation.

If difficulty with either mask ventilation or tracheal intubation is expected, then, according to the ASA Difficult Airway Algorithm, intubation and extubation should be performed while the patient is awake [1].

Rapid sequence induction maybe considered in obese and sleep apnea syndrome patients, with symptomatic gastroesophageal reflux or other predisposed conditions such as diabetes mellitus and gastrointestinal conditions, as there is a high chance of reflux resulting in aspiration [2].

If tracheal intubation is to be done using a flexible fiberscope while the patient is awake, it is essential that the patient is properly prepared by topical and nerve block anesthesia of the upper airway.

If intubation is to be done with the patient asleep, the patient should be fully preoxygenated because an obese patient with a relatively small functional residual capacity (FRC) and high oxygen consumption desaturates much more rapidly during obstructive apnea than a normal patient [3].

11.4 Extubation

The algorithm for extubation must be designed based on the surgical procedure performed and the condition of the patient. Although in most cases, it is preferable to extubate in a fully awake patient.

Full recovery from neuromuscular blockade should be proven using a neuromuscular blockade monitor and a sustained head lift for 5 seconds.

Extubation in the reverse Trendelenburg or semi-upright position minimizes the compression of the diaphragm by the abdominal contents.

11.5   REM Sleep Rebound

OSA patients during the postoperative period show highly fragmented sleep patterns for 1–2 days with a significant reduction of REM sleep [4].

This is followed by an increase in the amount of REM sleep [Rebound] during the 3rd to 5th postoperative nights. This can cause hypotonia and unstable breathing leading to hypoxemia. It can also be associated with tachycardia, hemodynamic instability, and myocardial infarction [4] (Table 11.2).

11.6   Postoperative Monitoring

Patients with OSA are prone to have respiratory and cardiovascular (hypertension, arrhythmia, myocardial ischemia, and infarction) complications in the postoperative period. The use of continuous airway pressure, preoperatively and postoperatively, would help in reducing the risk of complications.

Continuous positive airway pressure (CPAP) should be applied if the airway obstruction is persistent despite proper positioning of the patient and nasopharyngeal airway.

An adequate postoperative analgesia is an integral part of the anesthetic plan. Opioids are avoided as opioid induced upper airway obstruction is quite a common complication. Sedation and narcotic-based analgesia may exacerbate symptoms of sleep apnea resulting in respiratory depression and respiratory arrest in certain patients.

The use of non-steroidal anti-inflammatory drugs and local anesthetics for incision infiltration can minimize the necessity for the administration of large doses of narcotic drugs to achieve adequate analgesia (Table 11.3).

11.6.1 Keys to Anesthetic Management of OSA Surgeries

- It is mandatory to have a proper preoperative evaluation for every patient with OSA
- Anticipate difficult intubation in these patients as they are most often obese with a narrow oropharyngeal inlet
- Check for co-morbidities
- Whenever possible, an awake intubation is better as it reduces the risk
- It is recommended to reduce the duration of surgery and thus decrease surgical stress in patients undergoing OSA surgeries
- Avoid long acting sedatives and narcotics
- Expect violent/combative emergence
- Do not extubate when the patient is combative
- Extubate only when the patient is fully conscious
- Use nasopharyngeal airway after extubation
- Postoperatively consider NSAIDs over opioids for analgesia
- Consider PAP therapy in the postoperative period as well

References

1. Apfelbaum JL, Hagberg CA, Caplan RA, Connis RT, Nickinovich DG, Benumof JL, et al. Practice guidelines for management of the difficult airway: an updated report by the American Society of Anesthesiologists task force on management of the difficult airway [Internet]. Anesthesiology. 2013;118:251–70. American Society of Anesthesiologists. [cited 2021 Mar 14]. Available from: http://links.lww.com/ALN/A902.
2. Freid EB. The rapid sequence induction revisited: obesity and sleep apnea syndrome [Internet]. Anesthesiol Clin North Am. 2005;23:551–64. [cited 2021 Mar 14]. Available from: https://pubmed.ncbi.nlm.nih.gov/16005830/.

3. Klowden AJ, Nimmagadda U, Salter B. Perioperative and anesthesia management. In: Friedman M, editor. Sleep apnea and snoring. Philadelphia: Elsevier; 2009. p. 96–103.

4. Vasu TS, Grewal R, Doghramji K. Obstructive sleep apnea syndrome and perioperative complications: a systematic review of the literature [Internet]. J Clin Sleep Med. 2012;8(2):199–207. American Academy of Sleep Medicine. [cited 2020 Oct 4]. Available from: https://www.ncbi.nlm.nih.gov/pmc/articles/PMC3311420/?report=abstract.

The treatment aim of any OSA therapy is to control the symptoms and minimize its long-term morbidity by reducing the frequency of apneas and hypopneas.

As per AASM, the desired outcome of treatment includes the resolution of the clinical signs and the symptoms of OSA and the normalization of sleep quality, AHI, and oxyhemoglobin saturation [1].

OSA is not defined solely by one parameter; the diagnosis and management of this condition takes into account the patient symptomatology as well as the severity of the disease.

The definition of surgical success is more than just AHI reduction alone. Other outcomes like improvement in quality of life, improvement in sleep pattern, decreased day time sleepiness, and decreased headache should also be included in the postoperative assessment done to assess surgical success.

A surgical responder should not only aim at a reduction in AHI by 50% of the preoperative value but also aim at the resolution of other patient's others symptoms as observed by the patient or the patients bed partner, which will improve the patient's quality of life [2].

Kenny Pang et al proposed an acronym SLEEP GOAL [3], as a more comprehensive set of success parameters (Table 12.1):

S: Snoring visual analog scale [VAS]—based on descriptions from their spouse or bed partner,

Table 12.1 Success parameters (SLEEP GOAL)

Success parameters	
S	**Snoring VAS**—improvement in VAS by five points
L	**Latency of sleep onset (PSG or MLST)**—normalization of sleep latency (if it was abnormal pre-treatment), and/or improvement/normalization of the MSLT
E	**Epworth sleepiness scale**—normalization to less than 10 (if it was abnormal pre-treatment), or a reduction by five points
E	**Execution time**—improvement by more than 50%, using performance vigilance testing
P	**Pressure (SBP)**—(a) reduction in mean blood pressure by 7 mmHg, or (b) single reduction in either SBP or DBP by 10 mmHg or (c) 5 mmHg reduction in both
G	**Gross weight/BMI**—loss of >10% gross weight, and/or reduction of BMI from one category to another (by four points)
O	**Oxygenation**—improvement of duration (min) of O_2 <90% by at least half
A	**AHI via sleep study**—reduction by 50% and AHI <20
L	**Life score (PSQI)**—improvement in a relevant OSA related QOL score (i.e., PSQI or SF36 or FOSQ)

the severity of patients snoring is assessed using a VAS—of 10 points with 0 being (no snoring) to 10 (very severe snoring, bed partner leaves the room).

L: Latency of sleep onset (PSG)—It is considered an objective measurement of excessive daytime sleepiness (EDS). The Median sleep latency test [MSLT] consists of 4–5 naps of 20-min duration every 2 h during the day. The latency to sleep onset for each nap is averaged to determine the daytime sleep latency.

E: Epworth sleepiness scale—normalization to less than 10 (if it was abnormal pretreatment), or a reduction by five points

E: Execution time—improvement by more than 50%, using performance vigilance testing. The PVT is a sustained visual vigilance/attention test used to measure behavioral alertness. The PVT was presented on a computer screen and consisted of a series of 100 images of a white dot on a black screen visible for 50 ms with a random interstimulus interval of 3–7 s. The entire block lasted ~7 min. Subjects were instructed to press a button when the stimulus appeared on the screen as fast as they could while still maintaining accuracy. The reaction time and number of accurate responses are calculated.

P: Pressure (SBP)—(a) reduction in mean blood pressure by 7 mmHg, or (b) single reduction in either SBP or DBP by 10 mmHg, or (c) 5 mmHg reduction in both

G: Gross weight/BMI—loss of >10% gross weight, and/or reduction of BMI from one category to another (by four points)

O: Oxygenation—improvement of duration (min) of O_2 <90% by at least half A: AHI via sleep study—reduction by 50% and AHI <20

L: Life score (PSQI)—improvement in a relevant OSA related QOL score (i.e., PSQI or SF36 or FOSQ)

References

1. Epstein LJ, Kristo D, Strollo PJ, Friedman N, Malhotra A, Patil SP, et al. Clinical guideline for the evaluation, management and long-term care of obstructive sleep apnea in adults. J Clin Sleep Med [Internet]. 2009 Jun 15;5(3):263–76. [cited 2020 Oct 4]. Available from: https://www.ncbi.nlm.nih.gov/pmc/articles/PMC2699 173/?report=abstract.
2. Kezirian EJ, Weaver EM, Criswell MA, De Vries N, Woodson BT, Piccirillo JF. Reporting results of obstructive sleep apnea syndrome surgery trials [Internet]. Otolaryngol – Head Neck Surg. 2011;144:496–9. NIH Public Access. [cited 2020 Oct 4]. Available from: https://www.ncbi.nlm.nih.gov/pmc/articles/PMC5951288/?report=abstract.
3. Pang KP, Rotenberg BW. The SLEEP GOAL as a success criteria in obstructive sleep apnea therapy [Internet]. Vol. 273, European archives of oto-rhino-laryngology. Berlin: Springer Verlag; 2016. p. 1063–5. [cited 2020 Oct 4]. Available from: https://link.springer.com/article/10.1007/s00405-016-3944-2.

Obstructive sleep apnea (OSA) is one of the most common causes of sleep-disordered breathing (SDB) in children.

Children at risk need to be identified, investigated, and treated in a timely manner because of its long-term effects on neurocognitive, cardiovascular, and metabolic systems.

The adverse consequences of pediatric OSA may not be confined to the child's immediate well-being and development but these children may continue to become snorers and patients with OSA in their adulthood.

Habitual snoring which is an indicator of increased upper airway resistance is frequent occurrence in childhood especially among preschool and school aged children.

Successful management of SDB in children depends on the accurate identification of the site of obstruction and the assessment of severity of obstruction. Only then an appropriate surgical or non-surgical remedy maybe considered.

13.1 As per American Academy of Pediatrics: Spectrum of Pediatric Obstructive SDB in Increasing Order of Severity Encompasses [1]

1. *Primary snoring*—the mildest and most prevalent manifestation, which is defined as habitual snoring for more than 3 nights per week without apneas, hypopneas, frequent arousals, or gas exchange abnormalities;
2. *Upper airway resistance syndrome (UARS)*—comprises snoring, increased work of breathing and frequent arousals, without recognizable obstructive events or gas exchange abnormalities;
3. *OSA syndrome* manifests with recurrent events of partial or complete upper airway obstruction (hypopneas, obstructive or mixed apneas) with disruption of normal oxygenation, ventilation, and sleep pattern.

13.2 Levels of Obstruction

Etiology of pediatric OSA is broadly classified into

- conditions which result in intrinsic upper airway narrowing [Obstructive causes commonly due to adenotonsillar hypertrophy].
  - Level 1—Nose or nasopharyngeal
  - Level 2—Oropharyngeal
  - Level 3—Tongue base
  - Level 4—Supraglottic and glottic obstruction.
- and those that result in increased upper airway collapsibility, which could be due to loss of tone in conditions like cerebral palsy, neuro-

muscular disorders, or inflammatory conditions affecting the upper airways, such as allergic rhinitis and asthma.
- craniofacial syndromes resulting in upper airway narrowing such as micrognathia, macroglossia, and midface hypoplasia are often seen in pediatric population.

It can also be classified as

1. *Sleep-related breathing disorders in neonates and infants*
   - Congenital causes like nasal aplasia, stenosis, or atresia
   - Nasal or nasopharyngeal masses
   - Craniofacial anomalies in syndromic children who have hypoplastic maxilla and hypoplastic mandible like Treacher Collins syndrome, Pierre Robin syndrome
   - Macroglossia who could be seen as an association with syndromes or non-syndromic where there is muscular or lymphoid hypertrophy of tongue base.
   - Vascular malformations of tongue and pharynx
   - Neuromuscular disorders causing decreased tone.
2. *Causes of SDB in toddlers and older children.*
   - Rhinitis, nasal polyposis, and septal deviation
   - Nasopharyngeal stenosis in syndromic children like Down syndrome, Hurlers syndrome or iatrogenic post adenoidectomy.
   - Adenotonsillar hypertrophy
   - Obesity
   - Macroglossia
   - Vascular malformations and neuromuscular disorders.

13.3 Pediatric OSA Is Associated with

- *Inflammation*—There is emerging evidence that OSA is a disease with chronic low-grade systemic inflammation and increased oxidative stress [2]. At the nose, nasal nitric oxide (NO), a marker of airway inflammation, is elevated in children with OSA and primary snoring compared with healthy controls and this chronic low-grade inflammation can be associated with various long-term organ morbidities [2].
- *Neurocognitive and behavioral comorbidities*
  OSA in children is associated with behavioral problems or attention deficit hyperactivity disorder (ADHD) [2]. Even mild OSA and habitual snoring have been associated with hyperactivity, difficulty in concentrating, attention problems, and impulsivity. OSA in children is associated with hyperactivity, aggressive behaviors, lower social competencies, poor communication, and/or diminished adaptive skills [2].
- *Cardiovascular comorbidities*
  The most severe cardiovascular consequence of OSA is pulmonary hypertension, and the resultant cor-pulmonale if the OSA is left untreated. Children with OSA have also been shown to have diminished cardiac output and oxygen consumption at peak exercise capacity [2].
- *Sleep disturbances:*
  In children, sleep fragmentation often manifests as hyperactivity, difficulties in concentrating, and irritability [2]. In contrast to adult patients with OSA who have excessive daytime sleepiness, it is often a less common symptom in children.
- *Nocturnal enuresis:*
  A higher prevalence of nocturnal enuresis has been reported in children with OSA. This may be due to the inhibitory effects of OSA on arousal responses to changes in bladder pressure [2].

13.4 Symptoms and Signs of OSA

Nocturnal symptoms—snoring, gasping, increased work of breathing, restless sleep, witnessed apneas, or mouth breathing are symptoms suggestive of OSA

Daytime symptoms—hyperactivity, difficulty concentrating/learning difficulties, behavioral difficulties, excessive daytime sleepiness, and moodiness.

Table 13.1 Differences between pediatric and adult OSA

Feature	Children	Adults
Presentation		
Age	2–6 year peak	Increased in elderly
Sex	Male = Female	Male > Female
Obesity	Few	Most
Tonsils and adenoids	Often enlarged	Rarely enlarged
Daytime somnolence	Less common than in adults but can be seen	Common
Sleep		
Obstruction	Obstructive or hypoventilation	Obstructive apneas
Sleep architecture	Usually normal	Decreased delta and REM sleep
Arousals with obstruction	May not be seen	At the end of each apnea
Treatment		
Surgical	Definitive therapy in most patients	Minority of cases with inconsistent results
Medical (PAP therapy)	In selected patients	Most common therapy

Clinical examination in OSA: Adenotonsillar hypertrophy, obesity, midface deficiency, macroglossia, or mandibular hypoplasia may strengthen the suspicion of OSA. The differences between pediatric and adult OSA are mentioned in the Table 13.1.

13.5 Diagnosis of OSA in Children

The evaluation protocol consists of

- BMI
- Complete head and neck examination with ENT examination.
- Cardiopulmonary examination to auscultate heart and lungs with X-ray chest and ECG.
- CT scan
- Cine MRI
- DISE
- PSG
- AUDIO AND VIDEO TAPING

The gold standard test for the diagnosis of obstructive SDB in children and assessment of its severity is an overnight, attended, in-laboratory PSG study [2].

It helps in objective diagnosis and assessment of disturbances in respiratory parameters and sleep patterns.

The AHI is the most commonly used PSG parameter for the quantification of SDB severity. It comprises the number of mixed, obstructive, and central apneas and hypopneas per hour of total sleep time.

13.5.1 Even a Single Apnea is Pathological in Children

Full PSGs are laborious and require in-hospital monitoring of the patient by skilled staff overnight, and subsequent scoring and analysis.

Differences between AHI on PSG between adults and children are given in the chart below (Table 13.2).

- Other differences include
- Oxygen desaturation under 92%
- More than one obstructive apnea per hour
- Elevations in ETCo2 measurements more than 50 mm of Hg for more than 9% of sleep time or a peak level greater than 53 mm of Hg [3].

When PSGs are not available, possible alternatives include:

Nocturnal oximetry studies: oximetry studies have a high specificity but low sensitivity in the diagnosis of pediatric OSA. Three or more clusters of desaturation events ≥4% and at least three desaturations to <90% are considered abnormal (McGill criteria) [2].

Table 13.2 Polysomnographic criteria for severity of OSA in pediatric Vs adult

OSA severity	Pediatric	Adult
Normal	0	<5
Mild	1–5	5–15
Moderate	6–10	16–30
Severe	>10	>30

Respiratory polygraphy (RP) studies: respiratory polygraphies are essentially PSGs without the EEG, EMG, and EOG sensors.

Home RP or PSG: there has been a recent trend towards performing ambulatory PSG, because they are less expensive alternative to in-lab PSGs, and the results represent the child's typical night's sleep at home.

Pediatric sleep questionnaire: this parent-filled questionnaire assesses symptoms of SDB, such as snoring, excessive daytime sleepiness, attention problems, and hyperactive behavior in children aged 2–18 years.

Sleep clinical record: this is a diagnostic tool composed of physical examination, subjective symptoms, and clinical history of behavioral and cognitive problems. These items are used to determine the sleep clinical score (SCS). A SCS of ≥ 6.5 is considered positive for OSA [4]. This may potentially be a useful tool to screen patients for suspected OSA (Tables 13.3, 13.4 and 13.5).

Table 13.3 Sleep clinical score

Sleep clinical score [4]		
ITEM 1	Signs of oral breathing	2 points
	Moderate/severe nasal obstruction and/or habitual nasal obstruction	2 points
	Septum nose deviation	2 points
	Tonsillar hypertrophy Grade III–IV	2 points
	Freidman palate position III–IV	2 points
	Dental/skeletal malocclusion	2 points
	Narrow palate	2 points
	Obese or adenoid phenotype	2 points
ITEM 2	Brouillette questionnaire ≥ -1 and/or	0.5 points
	Presence of other symptoms (at least one item) • Limb movements • Known EEG paroxysmal activity • Daytime somnolence • Cephalalgia • Enuresis • Nocturnal choking	0.5 points
ITEM 3	Positive ADHD rating scale	1 point
TOTAL SLEEP CLINICAL SCORE (SCS)		
A SCS ≥ 6.5 is considered positive for OSA		

Table 13.4 Brouillette Questionnaire

Brouillette questionairre/observations [5]	
D	Difficulty in breathing during sleep? 0 = Never; 1 = Occasionally; 2 = Frequently; 3 = Always
A	Stops breathing during sleep? 0 = No; 1 = Yes
S	Snoring? 0 = Never; 1 = Occasionally; 2 = Frequently; 3 = Always
BROUILLETTE SCORE = $1.42 \times D + 1.41 \times A + 0.71 \times S - 3.83$	
Score	Interpretation
>3.5	Diagnostic for OSA
Between -1 and 3.5	Suggestive for OSA
<-1	Absence of OSA

13.6 Treatment of OSA in Children

Individual risk factors predisposing for OSA, the presence of OSA-related co-morbidities, and the kind and severity of symptoms should determine the priority for treatment and the therapeutic strategy.

A stepwise treatment approach should be used until there is a complete resolution of the OSA. This may include a combination of different treatment modalities depending on severity and cause for the upper airway obstruction.

Weight loss if the child is overweight or obese. There is data supporting the efficacy of weight loss as a treatment in obese adolescents.

Nasal corticosteroids and/or oral montelukast: A 6 to 12 weeks course of nasal steroids and/or montelukast may reduce adenoidal size in children with mild to moderate OSA [2].

Adenotonsillectomy: In contrast to adults where PAP therapy is considered as a gold standard, surgery is the gold standard in the treatment of pediatric OSA and today adenotonsillectomy is the most effective therapy in children with OSA and adenotonsillar hypertrophy.

American Academy of Pediatrics (AAP) recommends adenotonsillectomy as the first-line

Table 13.5 Pediatric sleep questionnaire

Pediatric sleep questionnaire [6] While sleeping does your child…	Yes	No	Don't know
Snore more than half the time?			
Always snore?			
Snore loudly?			
Have "heavy" or loud breathing?			
Have trouble breathing or struggle to breathe?			
Have you ever…			
Seen your child stop breathing during the night?			
Does your child….			
Tend to breathe through the mouth during the day?			
Have a dry mouth on waking up in the morning?			
Occasionally wet the bed?			
Wake up feeling un-refreshed in the morning?			
Have a problem with sleepiness during the day?			
Has a teacher or other supervisor commented that your child appears sleepy during the day?			
Is it hard to wake your child up in the morning?			
Does your child wake up with headaches in the morning?			
Did your child stop growing at a normal rate at any time since birth?			
Is your child overweight?			
This child often…			
Does not seem to listen when spoken to directly			
Has difficulty organizing tasks			
Is easily distracted by extraneous stimuli			
Fidgets with hands or feet or squirms in seat			
Is "on the go" or often acts as if "driven by a motor"			
Interrupts or intrudes on others (e.g., butts into conversations or games)			
Total Number of "Yes" Responses =			

If eight or more statements are answered "yes," consider referring for sleep evaluation

treatment for children with adenotonsillar hypertrophy. Subtotal tonsillectomies, also known as tonsillotomies, have been gaining popularity in younger children and infants as they have lower postoperative complication rates [2].

13.7 Indication for Adenotonsillectomy in SDB

1. PSG documented OSA
2. Adenotonsillar hypertrophy associated with:
   (a) Cor-pulmonale
   (b) Failure to thrive
   (c) Dysphagia
   (d) Speech abnormalities
   (e) Craniofacial growth abnormalities
   (f) Occlusion abnormalities
3. For healthy children with the common presentation of SDB: somnolence, behavioral problems, poor cognitive performance, nocturnal enuresis, and a physical exam consistent with adenotonsillar hypertrophy, with or without witnessed apneas, it is reasonable to proceed with T&A without prior polysomnogram.

13.8 Contraindications for Adenotonsillectomy

1. Hemoglobin level less than 10g%
2. Presence of acute infection in upper respiratory tract

3. Children under 3 years of age
4. Overt or submucous cleft palate
5. Bleeding disorders, e.g. leukemia, purpura, aplastic anemia, hemophilia
6. At the time of epidemic of polio
7. Uncontrolled systemic disease, e.g. diabetes, cardiac disease, hypertension, or asthma.
8. Tonsillectomy is avoided during the period of menses.

13.9   Tonsillectomy Techniques

Cold steel method: The dissection technique is the most common method of cold steel tonsillectomy. In this technique, the tonsil is pulled medially and the mucosa overlying the tonsil capsule is incised. The dissection continues in the plane of loose areolar tissue between the tonsil tissue and the pharyngeal muscles using a dissector and the tonsil is excised completely.

Diathermy tonsillectomy: Bipolar dissection tonsillectomy is an alternative method to traditional cold steel tonsillectomy. This method is associated with reduced intraoperative bleeding but increased pain. Monopolar dissection is known to be associated with more postoperative pain than other techniques [7].

Coblation tonsillectomy: Coblation technology utilizes a system of radiofrequency bipolar electrical current that passes through a medium of normal saline, which results in the production of a plasma field of sodium ions. These energized ions are able to break down intercellular bonds and effectively vaporize tissue at a temperature of only $60°$ C. This vaporization theoretically results in effective dissection with less postoperative pain from thermal injury. The technique can be utilized for complete tonsillectomy or for intracapsular tonsillectomy [7].

Harmonic Scalpel: Harmonic scalpel utilizes ultrasonic technology to cut and coagulate tissues, resulting in minimal tissue damage from thermal trauma. The device converts electrical energy from a generator into mechanical vibration through a transducer that consists of piezoelectric ceramics, generating a back-and-forth vibration of the blade at a frequency of approximately 55.5 kHz. The device can cut tissue on low- and high-power settings and can also coagulate bleeding tissue [7].

Laser tonsillectomy: Using a laser as a tool to dissect out the tonsils has been claimed to have advantages in terms of reduced bleeding and postoperative pain, but studies have failed to confirm this [7].

Radiofrequency assisted tonsillectomy: Radiofrequency is another tool used for tonsillectomy. Its advantages include lesser temperature and lesser lateral heat generation as compared to laser and cautery. It also provides excellent hemostasis.

13.10   Adenoidectomy Techniques

Curette adenoidectomy: Conventional method of performing adenoidectomy. Curette maybe visualized using mirror or it may be done as a blind procedure. Disadvantages of a blind procedure with unpredictable bleeding, poor access to choanal adenoid, and risk of trauma to the Eustachian cushions.

Ablation adenoidectomy: When compared with curettage, ablative techniques are more precise, faster, and result in less blood loss. A malleable suction cautery is curved to the appropriate arc and introduced into the nasopharynx. Under direct vision, the adenoids are ablated, starting at the choanae and progressing inferiorly.

Powered instrument adenoidectomy: Microdebrider and coblation are currently widely used for removal of adenoids and have been shown to be effective, efficient, and associated with better hemostasis but these techniques are more expensive as compared to traditional methods.

Laser adenoidectomy: KTP laser is associated with a high risk of nasopharyngeal stenosis. This serious complication has not been reported in a small series using gold laser for adenoidectomy. It is not a preferred method due to high cost and associated adverse effects [8].

Coblation adenoidectomy: Coblation assisted adenoidectomy with endoscopic visualization enables selective and precise removal of adenoid tissue with no significant risk of recurrence. It is also associated with lesser intraoperative and postoperative bleeding.

Endoscopic adenoidectomy: The application of endoscopic technology with telescopes for visualizing adenoidectomy via a trans-nasal approach has been described. Powered instruments maybe used trans-nasally or trans-orally to remove the adenoids. Advantages of this technique include precise removal of the tissue immediately adjacent to the Eustachian tube [9].

Powered Trans-nasal Adenoidectomy: It should be reserved for superiorly situated adenoids that project into the nasal cavity or for when choanal obstruction persists that cannot be removed at the conclusion of standard transoral surgery. The patient is positioned as for endoscopic sinus surgery. A zero degree telescope is used to visualize the adenoids. The adenoidal tissue is then removed under direct visualization using microdebrider/coblation/suction diathermy. An advantage of this technique is the neutral position that the head and neck are maintained. This is important in patients with cervical instability such as in children with Down syndrome [9].

Partial adenoidectomy: Children with developmental palatal abnormalities, such as submucous cleft may still require adenoidectomy. In the past, in order to prevent velopharyngeal insufficiency and hyper-nasal speech in these patients, only the lateral portion of the adenoids was removed in these patients; however, results from this technique have not withstood the test of time. Presently, partial adenoidectomy involves removing the superior two thirds of the adenoid pad, leaving sufficient adenoid tissue to prevent velopharyngeal insufficiency [9].

13.10.1 Risk Factors for Residual OSA after Adenotonsillectomy: [2]

1. Obesity
2. Severe OSA pre-surgery with an AHI of >20
3. Children aged >7 years

4. High FTP score
5. Children with asthma
6. Craniofacial abnormalities (e.g., Pierre Robin syndrome)
7. Chromosomal abnormalities (e.g., trisomy 21)
8. Neuromuscular disease.

Families should be counselled that OSA may recur after initial postoperative improvement.

13.10.2 Postoperative Complications of Adenotonsillectomy [7]

1. *Pain:* Post-tonsillectomy sore throat is normal for at least 1 week and on an average return to school or work can take 1–2 weeks.
2. *Hemorrhage:* Postoperative hemorrhage is the most common serious complication of adenotonsillectomy. Bleeding can be intraoperative, immediately postoperative (within 24 hours), or delayed (after 24 hours).
3. *Postoperative airway obstruction and pulmonary edema:* Children younger than 3 years may develop edema of the tongue, nasopharynx, and palate leading to airway obstruction. Postoperative pulmonary edema may arise in patients with long-term upper airway obstruction related to adenotonsillar hypertrophy, often necessitating prolonged mechanical ventilation. Patients with a prolonged history of obstructive sleep apnea should be observed closely after surgery with pulse oximetry in a monitored setting.

Risk factors for pulmonary postoperative complications after adenotonsillectomy:
   (a) Children <3 years
   (b) Severe   OSAHS   documented   by polysomnography
   (c) Failure to thrive
   (d) Obesity
   (e) Cardiac compromise (Cor-pulmonale, RVH, High BP)
   (f) Downs syndrome
   (g) History of prematurity
   (h) Craniofacial abnormalities

(i) Neuromuscular diseases
(j) Chronic lung disease
(k) Sickle cell disease
(l) Nasal problems (septal deviation, turbinate hypertrophy)
(m) Adenoid hypertrophy
(n) Mallampatti 3-4
(o) Upper respiratory tract infection in previous 4 week
(p) Marked obstruction with inhalation induction
(q) Difficulty in breathing in recovery room.
4. *Velopharyngeal insufficiency:* Velopharyngeal insufficiency (VPI), or hypernasality, is a relatively unusual complication primarily related to adenoidectomy.
5. *Nasopharyngeal stenosis:* It may arise as a result of excessive cauterization with extensive mucosal destruction involving the nasopharynx, lateral nasopharyngeal wall, and superior tonsillar pillar along with excessive resection of posterior tonsillar pillar tissue. Surgical intervention is required to resolve this problem.
6. *Cervical spine complications:* A rare complication of adenoidectomy or tonsillectomy is atlantoaxial subluxation (Grisel's syndrome). Patients with Grisel's syndrome have decalcification of the anterior arch of the atlas and laxity of the anterior transverse ligament between the atlas and axis. This leads to complaints of stiff neck with spasm of the sternocleidomastoid or deep cervical muscle. Patients with Down's syndrome are more prone to it.

13.11 Lingual Tonsillectomy

10–20% of children have persistent OSA following tonsillectomy and adenoidectomy [10].

One of the more common overlooked sites for continued obstruction is lingual tonsil hypertrophy.

Upper airway obstruction involving the lingual tonsils is evaluated by awake flexible fiberoptic endoscopy, sleep/sedated fluoroscopy, sedated cine MRI, and intraoperative sedated endoscopy. MRI is able to distinguish between lingual tonsil tissue and base of tongue musculature [10].

Lingual tonsil hypertrophy resulting in sleep-disordered breathing or other symptomatic airway issues is an indication for lingual tonsillectomy.

Lingual tonsillectomy can be done using suction electrocautery, laser, microdebrider, or coblation.

Coblation   lingual   tonsillectomy
Radiofrequency lingual tonsillectomy

Rapid maxillary expansion or orthodontic appliances: several studies have shown that rapid maxillary expansion can be efficacious in the treatment of OSA in carefully selected patients [2].

It is beneficial as a treatment in children with OSA and non-syndromic craniofacial abnormalities [2].

13.11.1 CPAP or Non-Invasive Positive Pressure Ventilation (NIPPV) for Nocturnal Hypoventilation

Indications [2]:

1. Children who have residual OSA after adenotonsillectomy
2. OSA related to obesity, craniofacial abnormalities, neuromuscular disorders, those who do not have significant adenotonsillar hypertrophy, or those who choose not to undergo surgery

The goal is to maintain patency of the upper airway throughout the respiratory cycle, improve functional residual lung capacity, and decrease work of breathing. Starting CPAP in children can be challenging, a multidisciplinary team approach works best and parental involvement and education is crucial.

For most children with OSA, CPAP will be effective.

BiPap is indicated in children with other co-existing conditions such as neuromuscular disease, craniofacial syndromes, or obesity hypoventilation [2].

Complications of CPAP and BiPAP include nasal congestion, rhinorrhea, epistaxis, facial skin erythema related to the mask, discomfort from air leak, abdominal distension, and midface retrusion.

Tracheostomy, craniofacial surgery: craniofacial surgery has been shown to be successful in children with syndromic craniofacial abnormalities [2].

Tracheostomy has the highest efficacy in the treatment of obstructive SDB when compared to other surgical interventions but is associated with worse quality of life and psychosocial development [2].

In clinical practice, craniofacial surgery and tracheostomy are mostly reserved for the most severe cases when all other treatment options have failed [2].

13.11.2   Surgeries for Pediatric OSA

1. Nasal/nasopharyngeal surgery:
   - Septoplasty
   - RFRIT
   - Choanal atresia repair
   - Nasal Polypectomy

2. Oropharyngeal Surgery:
   - Tonsillectomy-Coblator or radiofrequency assisted
   - UPPP

3. Surgery for Macroglossia:
   - Radiofrequency channeling
   - Coblation channeling
   - Lingual tonsillectomy
   - Tongue suture suspension
   - Surgical tongue base reduction

4. Surgery for Larynx:
   - Laryngomalacia (LM) –

     The three main LM types are identified as follows [11]:

     Type I: Inward collapse of the aryepiglottic (AE) folds on inspiration

     Type II: Curled tubular epiglottis with shortened AE folds, which collapses circumferentially on inspiration

     Type III: An overhanging epiglottis that collapses

     Indications for surgery: Severe stridor with compromised airway, feeding difficulties, failure to thrive, and obstructive sleep [11].

     Surgeries for LM: Supraglottoplasty is done in type I and type II LM while epiglottopexy is done in type III LM [11] (Figs. 13.1 and 13.2).

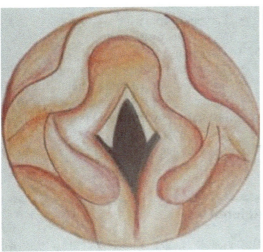 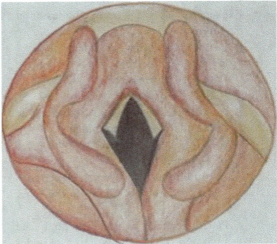

Fig. 13.1 Supraglottoplasty mucosal incisions

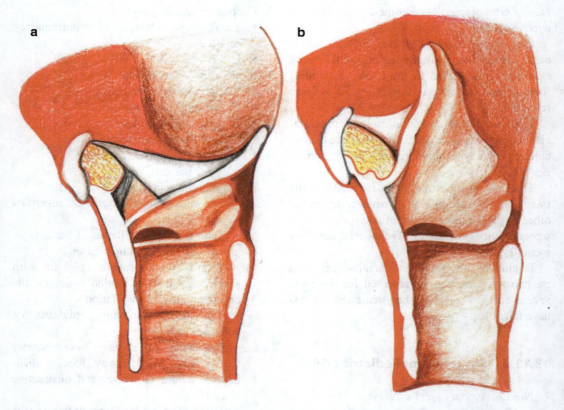

Fig. 13.2 Epiglottopexy for type III laryngomalacia. (**a**) Raw area is created on the tongue base and lingual aspect of the epiglottis (yellow arrows). (**b**) An epiglottopexy is performed, using 4.0 vicryl sutures to stitch the epiglottis to the tongue base with an endoscopic needle holder

- Laryngeal web excision
- Glottic and subglottic stenosis
- Excision of any space occupying lesion of the larynx
- Cordotomy for a bilateral abductor palsy
  - Posterior 1/3 to ½ of vocal cord along with vocal process removed laterally up to thyroid cartilage
  - A part of false cord may also have to be removed if they are prominent
  - Aim is to create a posterior glottic space of 4-5mm X 6mm
  - Depending on improvement sometimes the procedure is required on the other side
  - Patient requires to be taken for a 2nd time into OT for slough removal under GA for better results
  - Tracheostomy NOT required. Can be operated with endotracheal tube.

5. Surgeries for syndromic children:
   - Hypoplasia of midface and mandible
   - Labioglossopexy for glossoptosis
   - Mandibular distraction
6. Tracheostomy
   - Technique—"Starplasty" named for the fashion in which a circumferential tracheocutaneous fistula is created. This has to be maintained by traditional pediatric tracheostomy tubes
   - After the age of 12 yrs LTTF tracheostomy may be a viable option.

References

1. Gipson K, Lu M, Kinane TB. Sleep-disordered breathing in children. Pediatr Rev [Internet]. 2019 Jan 1;40(1):3–12. [cited 2020 Oct 4]. Available from: https://pedsinreview.aappublications.org/content/40/1/3.

2. Dehlink E. Update on paediatric obstructive sleep apnoea. J Thorac Dis [Internet]. 2016;8(2):224–35. [cited 2020 Oct 4]. Available from: www.jthoracdis. com.

3. Childhood sleep apnea workup: approach considerations, polysomnography, apnea hypopnea index [Internet]. [cited 2020 Oct 4]. Available from: https://emedicine.medscape.com/article/1004104-workup#c8.

4. Villa MP, Paolino MC, Castaldo R, Vanacore N, Rizzoli A, Miano S, et al. Sleep clinical record: an aid to rapid and accurate diagnosis of paediatric sleep disordered breathing. [cited 2020 Oct 4]. Available from: www.erj.ersjournals.com/misc/cmeinfo.xhtml.

5. Bannink N, Mathijssen IMJ, Joosten KFM. Can parents predict obstructive sleep apnea in children with syndromic or complex craniosynostosis? Int J Oral Maxillofac Surg. 2010 May 1;39(5):421–3.

6. Chervin RD, Hedger K, Dillon JE, Pituch KJ. Pediatric sleep questionnaire (PSQ): validity and reliability of scales for sleep-disordered breathing, snoring, sleepiness, and behavioral problems. Sleep Med [Internet]. 2000 Feb 1;1(1):21–32. [cited 2020 Oct 4]. Available from: https://pubmed.ncbi.nlm.nih.gov/10733617/.

7. Shirley WP, Woolley AL, Wiatrak BJ. Pharyngitis and adenotonsillar disease. In: Cummings otolaryngology – head and neck surgery. 5th ed. Missouri: Mosby; 2010. p. 2782–801.

8. J. Robb P. The adenoid and adenoidectomy. In: C. Watkinson J, W. Clarke R, editors. Scott-Brown's otorhinolaryngology and head and neck surgery Volume 1 [Internet]. 8th ed. CRC Press; 2018. p. 285–92. [cited 2020 Oct 4]. Available from: https://books.google.co.in/books?id=ODZlDwAAQBAJ&printsec=frontcover#v=onepage&q&f=false.

9. Discolo CM, Younes AA, Koltai PJ. Current techniques of adenoidectomy. Oper Tech Otolaryngol - Head Neck Surg. 2001 Dec 1;12(4):199–203.

10. Maturoa SC, Hartnick CJ. Pediatric lingual tonsillectomy. In: Pediatric airway surgery [Internet]. Basel: S. Karger AG; 2012. p. 109–11. [cited 2020 Oct 4]. Available from: https://pubmed.ncbi.nlm.nih.gov/22472240/.

11. Monnier P. Laryngomalacia (LM). In: Pediatric airway surgery [Internet]. Berlin: Springer; 2011. p. 99–106. [cited 2020 Oct 4]. Available from: https://www.google.co.in/books/edition/Pediatric_Airway_Surgery/xc7QJMquYLQC?hl=en&gbpv=1&dq=Supraglottoplasty+in+Suspension+Microlaryngoscopy&pg=PA101&printsec=frontcover.

14 Preventive Aspects in Obstructive Sleep Apnea

14.1 Breastfeeding Is Emerging as a Protective Factor Against Childhood Snoring

There has been increasing evidence of a preventive effect of breastfeeding on obstructive sleep apnea in children. It has been proven that the baby bottle deforms the dental arches, reducing sagittal mandibular growth.

Bottle feeding has shown to affect the development of the maxillary bone. Shorter the breastfeeding time, higher is the possibility that the child will develop malocclusion and narrow maxillary arch due to transverse maxillary deficiency (Figs. 14.1 and 14.2).

14.2 Early Diagnosis with Screening of Children to Prevent Them Transform into Adult OSAS

There are increased concerns for the growing concerns of pediatric OSA and obesity. Increasing evidence of obesity and its growing concerns to development of adult sleep apnea mandate a closer look at this disorder from primary prevention.

Primary prevention in terms of healthy habits, exercise, diet, and weight loss in obese children should be encouraged at the community level.

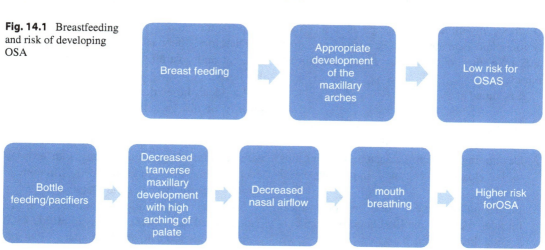

Fig. 14.1 Breastfeeding and risk of developing OSA

Fig. 14.2 Bottlefeeding/pacifiers and risk of developing OSA

D. S. Deenadayal, V. Bommakanti, *Management of Snoring and Obstructive Sleep Apnea*,
https://doi.org/10.1007/978-981-16-6620-9_14

Pediatricians must screen their outpatient patients for enlarged tonsil and adenoid and enquire with the parents for snoring or noisy breathing. When deemed necessary further testing and treatment must be encouraged.

Another potential site for early detection of OSA would be ENT clinics, where nasal septal deviation, enlarged tonsils/adenoids, and craniofacial abnormalities must be looked for and treated.

Screening must be done in allergy, immunology, and pulmonology clinics in those children presenting with breathing difficulties and primary pulmonary pathologies are considered and OSA is often overlooked.

Children and adolescent presenting with cardiac and neurological issue like stroke must also be primarily screened for OSA.

These measures decrease the probability of these children turning into OSA of adulthood. A healthy lifestyle with regular exercise associated with weight loss has been shown to reverse or improve OSA in selected patients.

Failed primary prevention would potentially increase the number of adulthood OSA.

14.3 Myofunctional Therapy in Prevention of OSAS

Orofacial myofunctional therapy is a series of isotonic and isometric exercises that strengthen and tone the tongue, lip, cheek, and throat muscles.

It is aimed at

1. Developing a good resting position of tongue by increasing the tone of the muscles.
2. Developing good lip occlusion, allowing lips to be closed at rest and improving nasal breathing.
3. Increasing the tone of oral and pharyngeal muscles reducing the likelihood of them collapsing during sleep.
4. Improving maxillary and mandibular skeleton framework allowing nasal breathing over mouth breathing.

The result of oral myofunctional therapeutic programs is the establishment of new neuromuscular patterns, correction of functional and resting postures, correction of chewing/swallowing/feeding patterns and thus decreases the probability of children getting into OSA of adulthood.

14.4 Biomarkers for OSA

OSA is often associated with dysfunctions in the metabolic and endocrine systems associated with chronic inflammation, hypoxemia, sleep fragmentation, and stress. The biomarkers which reflect the above condition are glycated hemoglobin (HbA1c), C-reactive protein (CRP), erythropoietin (EPO), and uric acid.

Unfortunately, the diagnostic utility of individual biomarkers or combinations of markers is inconclusive in confirmation of OSA but they when found elevated a strong suspicion for underlying OSA must be considered.

The prevalence of OSA is high (particularly with the obesity pandemic) and accurately diagnosing OSA is challenging and costly. Qualified sleep labs are not universally available resulting in delayed diagnosis.

Home sleep study although has become freely available and acceptable, misses arousals and sleep fragmentation.

Therefore, there is a need to develop more efficient and cost-effective approaches to OSA diagnosis.

An ideal biomarker should correlate with severity of disease and also indicate treatment response.

The biomarker should help differentiate cases with recurrent hypoxemia versus with arousal/sleep fragmentation only and help differentiate between obstructive and central apnea.

A recent study by Ambati et al in 2020 on 713 patients used the SomaScan array to profile 1300 proteins to identify novel sleep apnea biomarkers, and to develop multivariate constructs to predict sleep apnea phenotypes based on proteomic profiles.

Obstructive sleep apnea was associated with 65 proteins, predominantly modulating complement and coagulation pathways, while central apnea was associated with ROBO3 and cystatin F proteins. Their study identifies proteomic signatures and associated biological pathways in sleep apnea.

Multiplex protein assays offer diagnostic potential and provide new insights into the biological basis of sleep-disordered breathing.

Newer Technological Tools in Obstructive Sleep Apnea

15

15.1 Radiofrequency in Snoring and OSA

Radiofrequency is a novel surgical modality employing a temperature energy source of 4.0 MHz high-frequency radio waves. It is a completely different modality from electrocautery and laser.

There are numerous advantages of radiofrequency like precise bloodless surgery, hemostasis, debulking, tissue ablation, and vaporization. The results are attributable to the decreased risk factors and increased safety to the patient and medical personnel involved.

15.2 Mechanism of Action

Radio waves are high frequency, low voltage waves which have a power of 140 W. These radio waves are transmitted from a radiofrequency electrode to the target tissue [1].

The targeted tissue/cells absorb the energy due to high water content. Their absorption causes intracellular fluid to boil leading to cell wall expansion, leading to explosion—this process is called volatilization.

Volatilization results in cell conversion to vapor, also emitting low temperature steam that

aims at coagulation of tissue. There is minimum lateral heat generation hence avoiding tissue damage on the adjacent sides.

Since there is minimal charring of tissue, the scar heals faster and the operative site heals faster.

15.3 Radiofrequency Usage in Osahs

1. Tonsillectomy and adenoidectomy
2. Somnoplasty
3. Zeta pharyngoplasty
4. Expansion sphincter pharyngoplasty
5. Volumetric reduction of tongue base
6. For minor oropharyngeal procedures like uvulectomy.

15.4 Coblation in OSA Surgeries

Coblation is a relatively new, low-temperature electrosurgery technique that has multiple applications in ENT and head neck surgery.

Coblation is short for "Cold ablation/controlled ablation." It uses an ionized plasma field as a surgical tool for cutting and coagulating tissues.

Table 15.1 Comparison between radiofrequency, coblation, and electrocautery as a tool in OSA surgeries

	Radiofrequency	Coblation	Electrocautery
Temperature	55–65 °C	40–70 °C	>400 °C
Thermal penetration	Minimal	Minimal	Deep
Effects on target tissue	Minimal lateral heat generation and thus adjacent tissue charring is minimal.	Gentle removal/ dissolution	Rapid heating/burning and charring
Effects on neighboring tissue	Minimal	Minimal damage	Substantial damage
Better tool for stiffening procedure	Yes	Not an ideal tool	Can be used but not preferred.
Better tool for resection	Yes	Yes—Advantage of least blood loss	No

It is unique in that it utilizes RF energy to create a plasma field of ionized particles. A unique feature of this technology is that different coblation wands generate varying amounts of heat, and either ablate or volumetrically reduce the tissue. This gives the cobaltion a versatility for use in any surgical procedure.

15.4.1 Mechanism of Action

Coblation operates at low frequency [100 kHz] and low voltage [100–300 V] and employs a conductive fluid usually isotonic saline between the electrodes. There are two electrodes, active and return electrode. When an electric voltage is applied between the electrodes and saline flows—this saline is converted to ionized sodium ions or the plasma [2].

This ionized plasma do not travel far, as a result at the tissue level the molecular dissociation is very precise and the collateral damage is minimal.

The use of saline in this technique makes the temperature at tissue very low and thus helps to avoid charring and subsequent tissue damage. This technology can be helpful not just in cutting the tissue but also in cutting and coagulating the

tissue at the same time causing minimal blood loss in surgery.

15.4.2 Applications of Coblation in ENT

1. Turbinate reduction
2. Adenoidectomy
3. Tonsillectomy
4. Soft palate reduction
5. Tongue base reduction

15.5 Radiofrequency V/S Coblation V/S Electrocautery (Table 15.1)

References

1. Hong K, Georgiades C. Radiofrequency ablation: Mechanism of action and devices. J Vasc Interv Radiol [Internet]. 2010 Aug;21(Suppl. 8):S179–86. [cited 2021 Mar 14]. Available from: https://pubmed.ncbi. nlm.nih.gov/20656227/.
2. Shirley WP, Woolley AL, Wiatrak BJ. Pharyngitis and adenotonsillar disease. In: Cummings otolaryngology – head and neck surgery. 5th ed. Missouri: Mosby; 2010. p. 2782–801.

COVID-19 and Obstructive Sleep Apnea

16

The current COVID-19 pandemic has been a challenge, and especially for older adults, who are at a greater risk of complications from this disease.

With the ongoing pandemic, it is necessary to understand the factors that might predispose negative outcomes in COVID-19 patients. One of the predisposing factors for this is OSA. COVID-19 and OSA have been associated with increased risk of hospitalization, ICU admission, mechanical ventilation, and death.

The pandemic has not just increased the risk of COVID-19 infection in OSA patients but also with the implementation of lockdown there have been difficulties for patients and the doctors to screen, diagnose, and treat patients as they fall into the non-emergency category of treatment.

Going forward, a new normal must be set and newer methods for the diagnosis and treatment must be adapted. The principles on which it is based are the continuation of treatment, prioritizing treatment according to severity criteria, and the protection of patients and caregivers from possible viral transmission.

16.1 Similarities Between COVID-19 and OSA

The pathogenesis of OSA and COVID has striking similarities,

- OSA and COVID-19 are both pro-inflammatory states.
- It has been strongly argued that the culprit severe acute respiratory syndrome coronavirus-2 enters cells through angiotensin converting enzyme-2 receptors. Obesity is associated with an increased expression of these receptors in adipose tissue. It follows that infectivity would be more pronounced in obese OSA patients.
- Cardiac complications in COVID-19 and OSA are more or less similar which include hypertension, arrhythmias, heart failure, myocarditis, acute myocardial infarction, heart failure, and acute cardiac syndromes.
- In COVID, hypoxemia and altered hemodynamic status can precipitate a pro-coagulant state, which could further accentuate COVID-19 related coagulopathy.
- OSA is associated with increased risk for pulmonary embolism due to elevated D-Dimer lever, when associated with COVID-19 the risk further increases.

These findings suggest OSA as a risk factor for poor outcomes in patients hospitalized with COVID-19.

16.2 The Effects of Lockdown and Home Isolation

The implementation of lockdown measures and the massive surge in patients suffering from serious forms of COVID-19 infections has led to a reorganization of healthcare in many countries around the world. The focus has shifted to emergency treatment and the postponement of non-priority treatments.

OSAS is considered to be a non-emergency disease, hence its consequences can be serious, especially in the presence of specific comorbidities.

Lockdown and home isolation are causing grievous impact on the lives of people. Inability to go out and perform daily exercises or routines, decreased physical activity, work from home culture being promoted are further increasing the sedentary life style and further worsening OSA.

Reduced light exposure, reduced time outdoors, and increased exposure to light-emitting electronics might also contribute to poor sleep quality and alterations in the sleep–wakefulness cycle.

Social isolation, home confinement, anxiety, fear of getting infected, stress, and economic uncertainties due to the current COVID-19 pandemic directly impact sleep, promoting circadian disruption and acting as precipitators of insomnia.

Among older adults, loneliness seems to be an important additional factor.

16.3 The Way Forward

Telemedicine has evolved exponentially in last few months with the ongoing pandemic. This can be utilized very effectively in screening, diagnosis, and treatment for patients without a prior history of sleep-disordered breathing. In patients who have been already diagnosed with sleep-disordered breathing follow-up consultation or second opinions can be effective done with the telemedicine.

Telemedicine can be valuable in some pediatric patients, with the aid of their caregivers.

16.3.1 Virtual History and Physical Examination

Video calls can be an effective tool for eliciting history in patients who present with symptoms of OSA. The patients can be asked to fill the questionnaires prior to the consultation and keep record of physical parameters like height, weight, BMI, and neck circumference ready which help the clinician in the diagnosis.

The physical examination is a vital part of evaluating and providing treatment recommendations when assessing patients. Virtual medicine presents significant challenges for a meaningful physical examination.

The consulting physician and patient should understand that a virtual examination cannot replace a traditional examination, and that decisions leading to surgical intervention will require an in-person examination.

The virtual OSA directed physical examination should be performed methodically and efficiently, which begins with good lighting. Lighting can be optimized with a few simple tools available to most patients, including a flashlight and an improvised tongue depressor.

In combination with polysomnographic data, the physical examination findings can be surprisingly effective in screening patients with OSA.

However, evaluation of children may also be limited by their ability to cooperate with the examination.

A polysomnography must be considered in patients with high risk of OSA on initial video consultation and examination.

Thorough protective measures like sanitizing the instrument, maintain distance, use of protective masks, etc., must be taken by the technician involved in performing home sleep study as there is risk of transmission of infection from the technician to the patient and vice versa.

If on polysomnography the test is suggestive of severe OSA, recommendation for titration with CPAP or BiPAP may be tried and if the patients seek alternative form of treatment, then non-surgical modalities like mandibular advancement devices and tongue retaining devices must be offered.

If a surgical treatment is deemed necessary, then a risk versus benefit of the treatment modality must be thoroughly explained to patient and standard COVID-19 precautionary measures must be followed if a surgery is being performed.

For those patients diagnosed as mild or moderate OSA on a polysomnogram, conservative lifestyle measures like weight loss, prosthodontic devices must be advised.

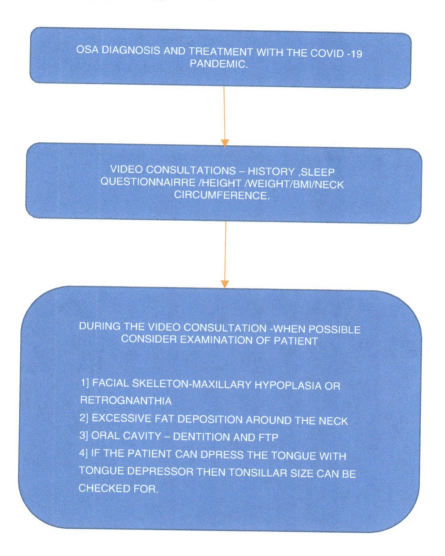

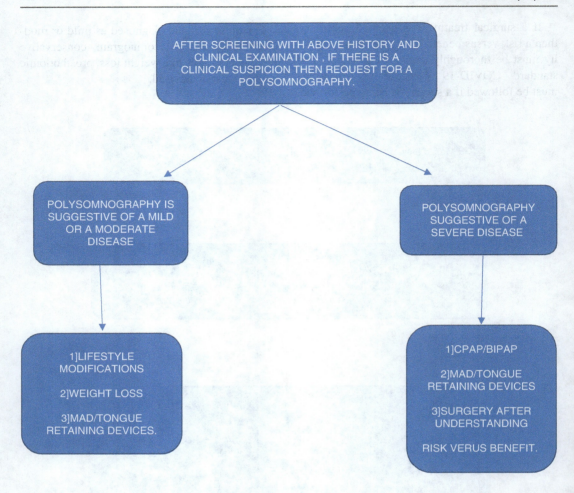

Medicolegal Aspects and Consent for OSA Surgeries

17

17.1 What Is a Consent?

A consent is an agreement where two or more parties agree to the same thing.

17.2 What Should a Consent for Sleep-Disordered Breathing Surgery Include?

The consent should be elaborate and should explain the following

1. Cause of the patient's snoring and sleep apnea.
2. The findings of the sleep study showing an abnormality in various parameters associated with snoring and obstructive sleep apnea such as AHI, RDI, flow limitations, etc.
3. An explanation to the patient regarding all the available alternate forms of therapy such as lifestyle modification, weight reduction, use of oral appliances, and positive airway pressure therapy [PAP] therapy.
4. It should also explain the sites of obstruction, whether only nasal/palatal/tongue base or a multilevel obstruction.
5. The consent should describe the aim of surgery—which is to either correct, remove, or reshape the tissue.

6. It should explain the various possible surgical complications—like change in voice/difficulty in swallowing/feeling of a lump in the throat and other complications depending on the type of surgery performed.
7. It should explain that there may be a need for a revision surgery if the current planned surgery does not help achieve the optimal success.
8. It should be documented that there may be a need for prolonged postoperative stay in the ICU, and in certain situations there may be a need for prolonged intubation and tracheostomy.
9. It should explain the long-term success of the procedure. It is most often anticipated that there are high chances of observing an improvement in the symptoms of snoring and OSA. Having said that, there is also no guarantee that it will be eliminated completely.
10. Any tissue or body part that is removed maybe sent for HPE or disposed of based on the doctor's judgement.
11. They must also be explained that other unforeseen incidents unrelated to the surgery such as cardiovascular and cerebrovascular events may occur.
12. All of the above must be explained to the patients in their own language. They must

D. S. Deenadayal, V. Bommakanti, *Management of Snoring and Obstructive Sleep Apnea*, https://doi.org/10.1007/978-981-16-6620-9_17

also be given the time to think and they should be encouraged to take further consultations and/or a second opinion about the same.

13. If the patient is a foreign national or does not know the language and if an interpreter is used for the same, then the interpreter's attestation is a must.

14. The signature of the patient on the consent is necessary. In the case of the patient being a minor, the legal representative's signature is mandatory. This must be attested by 2 witnesses from the patient's side.

15. The consent must contain a concluding statement from the surgeon with his signature which states that he has explained everything to the patient.

16. In certain situations, there may arise a need to alter the surgical plan intraoperatively and in a such scenario, a "Carte Blanche" consent is taken by which the patient gives complete freedom to the surgeon to perform the necessary surgery which may be beneficial to the patient.

The operating surgeon must also briefly explain the possible anesthetic complications that may occur, although the anesthetist will take their own separate detailed consent.

17.3　The Anesthetic Consent Should Include

1. Preanesthetic checkup with its findings and if any of these findings would affect the surgery.

2. Since OSA is associated with various co-morbidities, a cardiac/endocrinological/pulmonological checkup with their certification for fitness for the procedure to be performed under anesthesia must be obtained.

3. The type of anesthesia that is going to be administered to the patient and the effect of various anesthetic drugs on the patient.

17.4　Additional Parts of Consent [To Be Taken whenever Necessary]

1. Consent to take pictures/videos for the purpose of medical research or educational purpose with the assurance to the patient that their identity will not be shared.

2. Consent for utilization of blood products if it seems necessary.

3. Consent to allow observers into the operation theater for the purpose of advancing medical education.

4. Consent to allow assistant doctors to either assist or perform the procedure.

17.5　There Are 6 "P" for a Consent

1. Purpose of the procedure.
2. Preparation
3. Procedure [Operative]
4. Post procedure
5. Possible complications
6. Predictable outcome

17.6　Counselling

Before taking a consent from the patient, proper counselling is necessary so that he/she thoroughly understands each part of consent and is willing to proceed further. The counselling must comprise.

Medical counselling Financial counselling Psychological counselling.

17.7　Medical Counselling

The patient's existing problem must be explained to them in detail—the cause of the problem, the purpose of the treatment, and the need for the procedure that is going to be performed. The success rate of the procedure and the other available alternate forms of therapy should also be discussed. The risks of the treatment along with the inherent risks due to patients preexisting illness or specific risks of the surgery must be discussed elaborately. The consequences of not undergoing the treatment also must be discussed.

17.8 Financial Counselling

The approximate cost of the entire treatment with a finer breakup must be explained in order to ensure that there is no conflict between the hospital and patient on financial grounds. A brochure of various charges must be maintained by the hospital so that there is complete transparency regarding finances. All things explained to the patient must be documented.

17.9 Psychological Counselling

It is very difficult for any patient to be mentally prepared for surgery. After having been briefed about the possible adverse outcomes, it is likely that some patients will develop certain psychological issues like depression, anxiety, etc. Hence proper psychological counselling helps ensure that the patient is, both physically and mentally, ready for the surgery.

Future in Sleep Medicine

18

Obstructive sleep apnea (OSA) is a highly prevalent condition that is a major risk factor not just for the patient himself but also for the bystanders, as it is a clear risk factor for motor vehicle accidents. Proper evaluation and treatment is thus essential in managing patients with obstructive sleep apnea.

The team involved in the management of patients with obstructive sleep apnea constitutes a general physician, pulmonologist, ENT surgeon, dental surgeon, neurophysician, anesthetist, maxillofacial surgeon, psychiatrist, bariatric surgeon, pediatrician, psychologist, social worker, and sleep technician.

To assure a tailor-made treatment for each patient with OSA, it is necessary to set up a SLEEP BOARD that would constitute doctors of various specialties mentioned above to provide a holistic approach in managing patients at an individual level.

18.1 Sleep Board Is the Demand of the Day!

- The question that arises here is, Who is qualified to become a part of sleep board?

18.1.1 To Qualify as SDB Specialist

Specialist with 5 years' experience after passing their post-graduation or have had 1-year clinical experience in Sleep Medicine.

Specialist who has dedicated at least one third of their practice for sleep medicine for 3 years or 25 percent of the clinical practice in the sleep medicine for 4 years.

18.2 Role of Sleep Board

The three main roles for a sleep board are.

1. Management of SDB.
   The role of sleep board is to discuss about each patient with OSA as to what is the most appropriate form treatment considering various physical, mental, emotional, and psychological needs of the patient.
2. Prevention and education of SDB.
   - To prevent SDB it is essential to screen general population for OSA Educating healthcare workers will help in early identification of these patients and thus prevent long-term morbidities associated with these patients.
   - It is essential to establish multiple sleep boards and certified programs to involve more clinicians in the diagnosis.

D. S. Deenadayal, V. Bommakanti, *Management of Snoring and Obstructive Sleep Apnea*,
https://doi.org/10.1007/978-981-16-6620-9_18

3. To make programs/fellowships for pediatricians, pulmonologist, otolaryngologist to enhance younger generations involvement in sleep medicine.

Something needs to change like.

1. Increased training and empowerment in the management of OSA in adult and pediatric pulmonary fellowship programs. As experts in breathing, pulmonologists are well equipped to manage sleep-disordered breathing and already have alliances with respiratory care practitioners.
2. Elimination of the requirement for board certification and accreditation. Although controversial, evidence suggests that non-specialist care is as effective and less expensive than specialist care for OSA.
3. Encouraging insurance companies and credit policies to allow the use of CPAP in patients by reimbursing them for the same.
4. Accredited sleep clinics for easy routine follow up of patients.
5. Increased training for generalist clinicians, including non-physicians, in the diagnosis and chronic management of symptomatic, uncomplicated OSA, similar to the approach currently implemented for other chronic medical conditions such as COPD or asthma.
6. Enhanced education around sleep and its disorders in medical schools and other levels of training.
7. Enhancing sleep training for medical students and residents and have a super-specialty course in sleep medicine.
8. If super-specialty course seems a longer option the Education requirements for pulmonary and critical care training must change to enhance sleep training. Incorporating sleep training as an additional year in their existing 3 year course so that they learn pulmonary/critical care/sleep medicine in 4 years, with clear commitment to learning all three disciplines within this time frame. Such approaches would allow adequate time for meaningful research in sleep and breathing, an area in need of young investigators.
9. Multi-institutional training programs across various institutes in the cities and also across

the world would allow those individual institutions who may not have a learned sleep faculty with expertise in sleep-disordered breathing to disseminate the knowledge to the colleagues and juniors. Such programs could provide remote mentoring, sharing expertise, encourage networking among junior members, and provide career development guidance to the trainees across multiple sites.

18.2.1 Is it Practical to Have a Sleep Board?

To have a successful management of SDB it requires legislation regarding

- SDB education.
- SDB and its association with Road traffic accidents.
- Sleep clinics at all major hospitals.
- Primary prevention—Screening by health care workers.
- To encourage a super-specialty in Sleep Medicine.
- Legislation and insurance companies treatment policies and reimbursement should be realistic and facilitate all modes of treatment of SDB.
- Unified sleep disorder association to formulate guidelines for education/prevention and management.

Successful outcomes to patients with sleep-disordered breathing can only happen when there is a team approach and everyone works on single patient to determine what is the best possible treatment for the said patient.

As majority of accidents are due to SDB diagnosed or undiagnosed, PSG should be made mandatory prior to issuing or renewal of driver's license by any mode of transport (road, rail, water, air).

Sleep board can become a reality only if a medicolegal law is attached to it, and that every patient undergoing treatment for the same must have an approval from the sleep board before initiating the therapy.

Case Discussions

19

19.1 Case I

A 52-year-old male presented with chief complaints of snoring, disturbed sleep, daytime sleepiness, and reduced concentration at work since 5 yrs. He had a past history of nasal surgery and tonsillectomy. On examination tonsils were absent and septum was central. Polysomnography was done which revealed severe OSA with an Ahi of 36. OSA events were 228, with longest duration of 59 sec, hypopneas were 39 with longest duration of 1.38 min, central apneas were 13 with 27 sec longest duration. Total snoring events were 2117. Lowest oxygen saturation was 77%. Doppler tongue base showed that lingual artery was approximately 1.7 cm deep from the surface on both sides and distance from midline was 1.5 cm on both sides.

Patient refused CPAP. Patient was taken up for zetapalatoplasty and coblation tongue base reduction.

Post op polysomnography was normal (Fig. 19.1).

19.1.1 Case Discussion

Persistence of symptoms despite previous surgery should alert the physician to look for other levels of obstruction, in this case it was the palate and the enlarged tongue base causing the airway obstruction.

Before taking up the patient for surgery, a CPAP trial should be given and refusal or non-compliance to CPAP therapy should be documented.

Zetapalatoplasty is indicated after a documented failure of CPAP trial and in cases of previous tonsillectomy. The goal of ZPP is to widen the space between the palate and the posterior pharyngeal wall, between palate and the tongue base and to either maintain or widen the dimensions of lateral pharyngeal wall. Hence it is useful in cases of moderate to severe OSA with concentric collapse.

Coblation tongue base reduction reduces the tissue at the base of tongue and increases the retrolingual space. It is very important to map the course of the lingual artery preoperatively to avoid injury to it.

19.2 Case II

A 53-year-old male k/c/o OSA was on CPAP since 3 yrs. He presented mainly with complaints of unfreshened sleep even on CPAP, disturbed sleep, decreased energy levels, and decreased concentration levels. He wanted to know if there is other treatment available as he was not comfortable with CPAP. On examination revealed deviated septum to right, hypertrophied turbinates, grade 1 tonsils, and FTP 3. FLP Scopy and dynamic MRI were done.

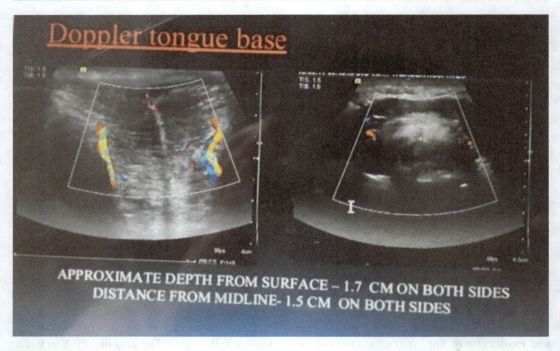

Fig. 19.1 Tongue base Doppler

Patient was taken up for zetapalatoplasty + septoplasty + inferior turbinoplasty + radiofrequency channeling of tongue base.

Postoperatively there was improvement in ESS and polysomnography parameters.

19.2.1 Case Discussion

Failure of CPAP therapy is an indication for surgical intervention in OSA.

Assessment of level of obstruction is important. This can be done through a thorough ENT and head and neck examination. Drug induced sleep endoscopy (DISE) can further help in assessing the type of palatal collapse, retrolingual space compromise, epiglottic collapse, and glottic airway. Direction of collapse can help in determining the type of palatal surgery that will benefit the patient. Degree of tongue base enlarged will also help in deciding whether the patient will benefit with a minimally invasive procedure or tongue base resection is required.

Dynamic MRI is an imaging modality that also helps in ascertaining the level of obstruction—retropalatal, retrolingual, or multilevel. Advantage of dynamic MRI is that it can provide a multiplanar dynamic view of the obstruction and aid in deciding the appropriate intervention.

Moderate to severe OSA usually involves multiple levels of obstruction in the collapsible upper airway as in this case. Multilevel pharyngeal surgery along with nose surgery (if nasal obstruction is significant), therefore, is usually required to surgically overcome the several sites of obstruction. There is no evidence of increased morbidity or complications with these procedures performed together.

19.3 Case III

A 35-year-old male presented with progressive severe cough, difficulty in breathing especially during inspiration, loss of concentration with daytime sleepiness, and sleep disturbances.

Work-up by a general physician resulted in diagnosis of chronic obstructive pulmonary disease
(COPD) with obstructive sleep apnea syndrome.
Patient was advised CPAP. There was no
improvement of symptoms, instead the symptoms worsened after using CPAP. Patient could
not tolerate CPAP. Patient was referred to us for
further management. His BMI was 24.22. ESS
was 9. Drug induced sleep endoscopy (DISE)
revealed a floppy epiglottis that was obstructing
the airway. Polysomnography showed severe
OSA.

   Patient was advised surgery.

19.3.1 Case Discussion

This case reinforces the importance of assessment of upper airway and the level of obstruction
before prescribing any therapy for obstructive
sleep apnea. In this case it was the floppy epiglot-
titis that was obstructing the airway during the
sleep.

   CPAP resulted in further aggravation of the
epiglottic collapse which is why the patient's
symptoms worsened and he was not able to tolerate the CPAP.

   Drug induced sleep endoscopy plays a key
role in the diagnosis of this condition.

   Epiglottic collapse is difficult to treat with
conservative therapies, such as oral appliances
and CPAP. Therefore, its identification has
important implications for surgical treatment.

   This patient underwent a partial epiglottectomy following which he was relieved of his
symptoms (Figs. 19.2 and 19.3).

19.4   Case IV

A 12-year-old male with no co-morbidities, came
with the complaints of temporal headaches,
mouth breathing, snoring, post nasal drip, nose
blocks, and decreased concentration levels. On
examination there was a spur to left, hypertrophied inferior turbinates, grade 3 tonsils, and
grade 3 adenoids (Figs. 19.4 and 19.5).

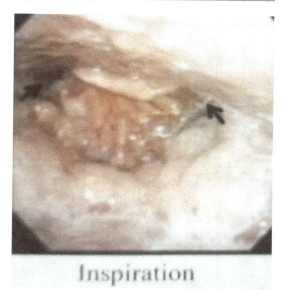

Fig. 19.2 Epiglottic Collapse

19.4.1 Case Discussion

Obstructive sleep apnea (OSA) is a common and
serious cause of morbidity during childhood.
Even mild OSA and habitual snoring have been
associated with hyperactivity, difficulty in concentrating, attention problems, and impulsivity.

   Adenotonsillar hypertrophy is the most frequent causative disease. In addition to it, nasal
allergy resulting in hypertrophied turbinates and
nasal obstruction can worsen the obstruction.

   Unlike in adults where the first line of treatment for obstructive sleep apnea, in pediatric
OSA surgical intervention in the form of adenotonsillectomy is the treatment of choice. Nasal
obstruction should also be addressed with turbinate reduction and minimal septoplasty to relieve
airway obstruction.

19.5   Case V

A 65-year-old male presented with complaints of
mild stridor and difficulty in breathing since
10 days. He had history of daytime somnolence
and breathlessness on exertion since 10 yrs.
Patient had visited pulmonologist and cardiolo-

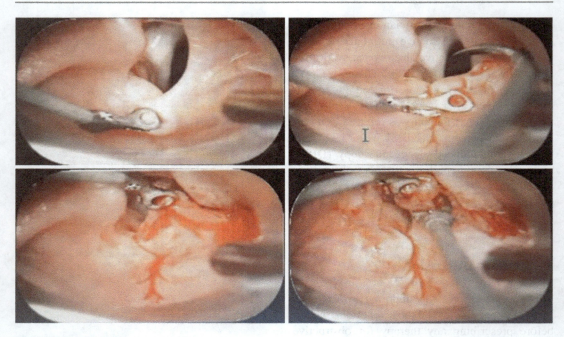

Fig. 19.3 Epiglottectomy

gist with above-mentioned complaints and was advised CPAP. Patient was not compliant for CPAP and had a stroke 4 yrs. back. On evaluation he was found to have bilateral abductor palsy with compromised glottic airway. This patient was taken up for posterior cordotomy under general anesthesia to create glottic airway. Postoperatively he was relieved of stridor and CPAP compliance also improved.

19.5.1 Case Discussion

Vocal cord paralysis is one of the rare causes of obstructive sleep apnea. Vocal cord palsy may develop as a result of trauma (surgical or non-surgical), inflammation, malignancy, neurological disorders or it may be idiopathic. In bilateral vocal cord paralysis, the glottic airway is com-

promised. In order to overcome the obstruction at the glottis, the patient creates a higher inspiratory pressure and hence dynamic compression occurs making inspiration more difficult.

Evaluation of OSA requires complete assessment of upper airway. Larynx is usually overlooked as a site of obstruction in OSA by many physicians. He was prescribed CPAP on the basis of sleep study. It was the laryngeal examination by an ENT surgeon that revealed the level of obstruction, that was otherwise missed. The compromised glottic airway made the patient intolerant to CPAP. Surgical intervention by posterior cordotomy not only improved the patient's symptoms but also improved his compliance to CPAP. Thus, an ENT consultation should always be taken in the multidisciplinary management of OSA patients to ascertain the level of obstruction and intervene surgically if needed to improve the upper airway patency.

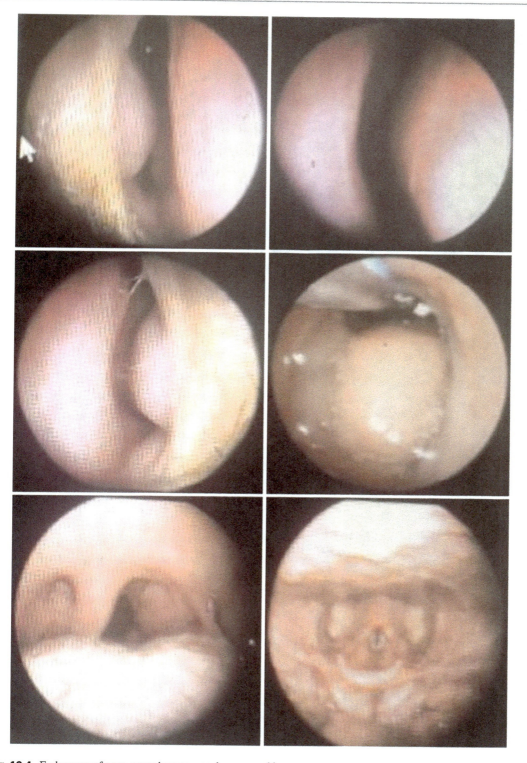

Fig. 19.4 Endoscopy of nose, nasopharynx, oropharynx, and larynx

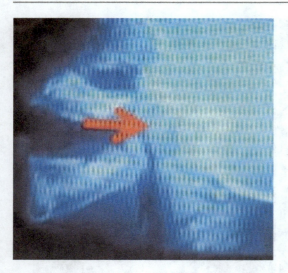

Fig. 19.5 X-ray nasopharynx showing grade 3 adenoid